Neurocritical Care

T0177325

Neurocritical Care

Edited by
Andrew M. Naidech
Northwestern University Feinberg School of Medicine, Chicago

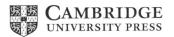
CAMBRIDGE
UNIVERSITY PRESS

CAMBRIDGE
UNIVERSITY PRESS

University Printing House, Cambridge CB2 8BS, United Kingdom

One Liberty Plaza, 20th Floor, New York, NY 10006, USA

477 Williamstown Road, Port Melbourne, VIC 3207, Australia

314–321, 3rd Floor, Plot 3, Splendor Forum, Jasola District Centre,
New Delhi – 110025, India

103 Penang Road, #05–06/07, Visioncrest Commercial, Singapore 238467

Cambridge University Press is part of the University of Cambridge.

It furthers the University's mission by disseminating knowledge in the pursuit of
education, learning, and research at the highest international levels of excellence.

www.cambridge.org
Information on this title: www.cambridge.org/9781108820868
DOI: 10.1017/9781108907682

© Cambridge University Press 2022

First published 2022

Printed in the United Kingdom by TJ Books Limited, Padstow Cornwall

A catalogue record for this publication is available from the British Library.

Library of Congress Cataloging-in-Publication Data
Names: Naidech, Andrew M., editor.
Title: Neurocritical care / edited by Andrew M. Naidech.
Other titles: Neurocritical care (Naidech)
Description: Cambridge, United Kingdom ; New York, NY : Cambridge
University Press, 2021. | Includes bibliographical references and index.
Identifiers: LCCN 2021025385 (print) | LCCN 2021025386 (ebook) |
ISBN 9781108820868 (paperback) | ISBN 9781108907682 (ebook)
Subjects: MESH: Central Nervous System Diseases – therapy |
Critical Care – methods | Intensive Care Units | BISAC: MEDICAL / Neurology
Classification: LCC RC350.N49 (print) | LCC RC350.N49 (ebook) |
NLM WL 301 | DDC 616.8/0428–dc23
LC record available at https://lccn.loc.gov/2021025385
LC ebook record available at https://lccn.loc.gov/2021025386

ISBN 978-1-108-82086-8 Paperback

Contents

Contributors

Michael L Ault, MD

Northwestern University, Department of Anesthesiology

Aimee Aysenne, MD, MPH

Tulane University, School of Medicine, Department of Clinical Neurosciences

Sherri A Braksick, MD

Mayo Clinic College of Medicine, Department of Neurology, Rochester, MN

Tiffany R Chang, MD

Department of Neurosurgery, University of Texas Health Science Center at Houston, Houston, TX

H Alex Choi, MD, MS

UT Health Neurosciences, McGovern Medical School, The University of Texas Health Science Center at Houston, Houston, TX

Charles L Francoeur, MD, MSc

Department of Anesthesia and Critical Care, CHU de Québec - Université Laval
Brandon Francis, MD, Department of Neurology, Michigan State University, East Lansing, MI

Kelsey Goostrey, BA, MPH

Clinical Research Coordinator, University of Massachusetts Medical School, Worcester, MA

Tyler Hinkel, MD
Northwestern Memorial Hospital

Ameeta Karmarkar, MD
Spartanburg Regional Medical Center, Spartanburg, SC

Swathi Kondapalli, MD
Northwestern University Feinberg School of Medicine, Department of Radiology

Alexander W Korutz, MD
Northwestern University Feinberg School of Medicine, Department of Radiology

Howard Lee, MD
Northwestern University Feinberg School of Medicine, Department of Radiology

Stephan A Mayer, MD
Director of Neurocritical Care and Emergency Neurological Services, Westchester Medical Center Health Network New York Medical College, Valhalla, NY

Deepika P McConnell, Pharm D, BCPS
Northwestern Medicine, Chicago, IL

Susanne Muehlschlegel, MD, MPH, FNCS, FAAN, FCCM
Departments of Neurology, Anesthesia/Critical Care and Surgery, University of Massachusetts Medical School, Worcester, MA

Andrew Naidech, MD, MSPH
Northwestern University, Feinberg School of Medicine, Department of Neurology, Chicago, IL

Alexander J Nemeth, MD
Northwestern University Feinberg School of Medicine, Department of Radiology

Peter Pruitt, MD

Northwestern University Feinberg School of Medicine, Department of Emergency Medicine

Alejandro A Rabinstein, MD

Mayo Clinic College of Medicine, Department of Neurology, Rochester, MN

Giang T Quach, DO

McGaw Medical Center of Northwestern University Feinberg School of Medicine

Martha Robinson, MD

Tulane University, School of Medicine, Department of Clinical Neurosciences

Eric J Russell, MD

Northwestern University Feinberg School of Medicine, Emeritus Chair of Radiology

Ahmed M Salem, MD MSc

Division of Pulmonary, Critical Care and Sleep Medicine, Department of Medicine, Baylor College of Medicine, Houston, TX

Michael B Shapiro, MD

Northwestern University Feinberg School of Medicine

Dionne E Swor, DO

Wake Forest University, Winston-Salem, NC

Muhammad Umair, MD

Northwestern University Feinberg School of Medicine, Department of Radiology

Tanuwong Viarasilpa, MD

Division of Critical Care, Department of Medicine, Siriraj Hospital, Mahidol University, Bangkok, Thailand

Introduction
The Practice of Neurocritical Care

Andrew M Naidech

"Good judgment is the result of experience and experience the result of bad judgment." – Mark Twain

Intensive care units exist for patients with severe disease, as well as for patients who are expected to be unstable. Unprovoked changes to vital signs, neurological examinations, laboratory results, and imaging are expected in such patients, although some events can be anticipated, rescued, or salvaged. One should know what comes next, how to communicate what has happened, and what is likely to happen next.

Being responsible for a neurological intensive care unit without knowledge and/or experience should provoke anxiety. This handbook is intended to improve your judgment from the experience of others. Each chapter has been authored by an expert in the field. We do not imply that there is no other way to manage neurologically critically ill patients, but only that this is one expert way to do so. Others may argue that there are better ways to manage specific problems, and, on occasion, it will be correct. However, the authors believe this book will not disappoint the clinicians in search of new knowledge, a refresher, and options.

Each chapter covers a crucial topic in neurological critical care (NCC). This does not mean this volume is exhaustive – there is always another topic that could benefit from its own explanation, another decision tree, and a refined protocol. Of note, this volume broadly excludes ischemic stroke, which is covered by another volume in this series. Exhaustion, however, is not the point. You need to know what to do in this shift on behalf of the patient and how to defend your actions the next time you round.

Blood pressure, temperature, heart rate, and respiratory rate are the classical vital signs. For patients with severe neurological disease, intracranial pressure (ICP) could be considered a fifth vital sign. Recognition and management of abnormal ICP are as important as managing the other vital signs and cannot take place without managing other vital signs. Dr. Stephan Mayer leads the reader through ICP interpretation and management, bringing a perspective honed over decades as a leading authority in the field.

Temperature dysregulation is common in NCC. Delicate neurologic mechanisms that are intended to maintain a normal temperature are frequently disturbed after severe neurological injury. Abnormal temperature is a consequence of neurologic injury, and it can make existing neurologic injury worse. However, some treatments of temperature dysregulation can be ineffective or worse. Understanding temperature dysregulation is important to interpret, predict, and manage temperature. Dr. Ameeta Karmarkar reviews the pathophysiology needed to understand temperature dysregulation and its effective management.

NCC is imaging-intensive. A working knowledge of neuroradiology is essential to diagnose, anticipate, and manage NCC patients. Neurologic diagnosis and management for both hemorrhagic (subarachnoid hemorrhage and intracerebral hemorrhage) and ischemic (particularly acute vessel occlusion) patients are authoritatively reviewed, led by Drs. Nemeth and Russell.

Critical care often comes with a need for a mechanical ventilator. Unfortunately, training in respiratory medicine is not always sufficient before starting in neurocritical care. Fortunately, Dr. Howard Lee provides instruction regarding management of the airway, oxygen, and mechanical ventilator.

Drug therapy for NCC is sometimes similar to that of other intensive care settings (e.g., antibiotics for sepsis) but is often peculiar to neurologic disease. Seizure medications, hypertonic fluids, and vasopressors to induce hypertension are uncommonly seen outside of a neurological intensive care unit. Like other intensive care units, a pharmacist is a strategic resource. Dr. Deepika McConnell reviews how to most effectively work with the most commonly used medications and the pharmacist, if you are fortunate enough to have one as a colleague. If you do not have a dedicated pharmacist, Dr. McConnell's level of expertise may help you convince your institution that the pharmacist is a crucial resource for patient care.

Intracerebral hemorrhage, bleeding into brain tissue, is the most morbid form of stroke. Early diagnosis and management of intracerebral hemorrhage can be lifesaving. Some patients require an acute therapy (e.g., blood pressure reduction, reversal of anticoagulant medication). Most patients require critical care management, which reduces complications and prepares the patient for the next phase of care (e.g., rehabilitation, nursing facility). Dr. Brandon Francis, a retired officer and a gentleman, reviews management of intracerebral hemorrhage.

Coagulopathy increases the likelihood of bleeding. Bleeding in the nervous system can quickly lead to permanent disability or death. Coagulopathy is complicated to measure once one gets beyond the prothrombin time and international normalized ratio. The diagnosis and management of coagulopathy are crucial to preventing death and disability in NCC. Dr. Tiffany Chang reviews measures of coagulation and how to correct disorders in the activation of coagulation, thrombosis, and fibrinolysis.

Subarachnoid hemorrhage, ruptured intracranial aneurysm, presents an unusual challenge. Typically, therapies for stroke are rescue therapies, for example, fibrinolysis after ischemic stroke. Patients with subarachnoid hemorrhage, however, may have two acute neurological changes. The first occurs at the time of aneurysmal rupture, and the second occurs about a week later with the heralding of symptomatic vasospasm. Dr. Alex Choi guides you through the diagnosis and management of subarachnoid hemorrhage.

Subdural hematoma has received less attention than intracerebral hemorrhage or subarachnoid hemorrhage. Yet, subdural hematomas will become more and more commonplace in an aging America that uses more anticoagulant medications for the prevention of vascular disease. Unlike intracerebral hemorrhage, subarachnoid hemorrhage, or neurotrauma, subdural hematoma has no grading scale, guidelines from randomized trials, or specifically approved treatment. Dr. Peter Pruitt fills the void on the diagnosis, assessment, and management of subdural hematoma.

Seizures and status epilepticus may occur without a precipitating condition and are a common complication of other neurological conditions, particularly intracranial hemorrhage or trauma. The longer seizures last, the worse the patient's outcome will be, so obliterating seizures quickly is crucial to maximizing patient outcomes. Dr. Swor reviews the management of status epilepticus in an intensive care setting.

Neurocritical Care takes place outside of dedicated neurologic units. Neurointensivists may be asked to provide consultation to evaluate coma and the likelihood of neurological recovery after coma generally, and cardiac arrest specifically. This condition has a long history of evaluation, complications (particularly myoclonic seizures), and prognosis. Drs. Braksick and Rabinstein update you on how to effectively evaluate and prognosticate after coma.

Many decisions will be yours to make; however, some of the most important decisions should be made in consultation. Decisions about goals of care, life-sustaining procedures (gastrostomy, tracheostomy), and do-not-resuscitate status should ideally involve the patient and/or a surrogate decision-maker. These conversations are often difficult, multilayered, and emotionally laden. Dr. Susanne Muehlschlegel, an expert in surrogate decision-making in NCC, leads you through best practices for these difficult conversations.

My colleagues and I have worked hard to compile this volume. We hope you find it useful and will share your feedback with us.

2

Intracranial Pressure Monitoring and Management

Tanuwong Viarasilpa, Charles L Francoeur, and Stephan A Mayer

Abstract

Intracranial hypertension is a life-threatening condition that if left unchecked can lead to brain herniation, cerebral ischemia, and brain death. Intracranial pressure (ICP) monitoring is frequently helpful for patient management. If placed, the monitor should be inserted in comatose patients at high risk for elevated ICP. ICP values, trends, and waveforms should be analyzed in conjunction with cerebral perfusion pressure (CPP) to guide therapy. Patients with elevated ICP can be managed using a tiered strategy that emphasizes cerebral spinal fluid drainage, sedation, and CPP optimization (tier one) prior to initiating bolus osmotherapy, hyperventilation, or paralysis (tier two). Multimodality monitoring therapy is a promising strategy that can detect secondary brain injury early and allow individualized treatment. Tier-three strategies for superrefractory ICP elevation include decompressive craniectomy, hypothermia, and pentobarbital infusion. Of these, craniectomy appears to be the most effective measure for reducing mortality, especially in younger patients.

2.1 Introduction

Intracranial pressure (ICP) is the pressure within the dura. In health, homeostatic mechanisms maintain ICP in a range from 3 to 15 mmHg (or 5 to 20 cm H_2O) in the supine position.[1] Elevated ICP is rapidly detrimental to brain function and can cause secondary cerebral ischemia and herniation. Treatment to restore ICP to normal must be given expeditiously, and it constitutes a cornerstone of acute care neurology.

2.2 Pathophysiology

ICP is determined by the volume within the cranial vault, which normally contains brain parenchyma (1,400 ml), cerebrospinal fluid (CSF, 150 ml), and blood within the cerebral vasculature (75 ml). If the volume of one component of the cranium increases, the others must decrease lest ICP will rise, a concept known as the Monro–Kellie doctrine. If the volume of brain parenchyma increases (cerebral infarction), excessive CSF accumulates (hydrocephalus), the cerebral vasculature excessively dilates (hyperemia), or a space occupying mass lesion develops, ICP will increase. At first, compensatory mechanisms will maintain ICP within the normal range because the system is compliant. CSF will be displaced out of the intracranial vault into the spinal axis, cerebral blood volume (CBV) will decrease as vascular beds are effaced, and brain tissue will be compressed. Once these mechanisms are exhausted, even small increments in intracranial volume can lead to dramatic increases in ICP as compliance is reduced (Figure 2.1). Intracranial hypertension, or "ICP crisis," is generally defined as a persistent elevation of ICP ≥20 mmHg for more than 10 minutes.[2,3] Common causes of intracranial hypertension are shown in Table 2.1.

2.2.1 CONSEQUENCES OF INTRACRANIAL HYPERTENSION

Intracranial hypertension is a common and treatable cause of secondary brain injury after traumatic brain injury (TBI) or massive stroke. A severe increase in ICP in one area of the brain can lead to compartmentalized pressure gradients and brain tissue shifting, a process called "brain

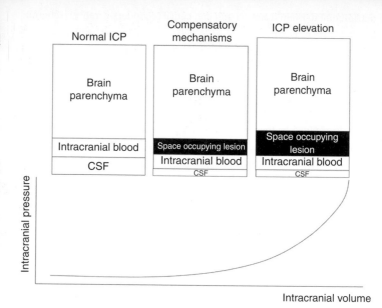

Figure 2.1 Compensatory mechanisms for preventing intracranial pressure (ICP) elevation. Compensatory mechanisms for preventing ICP elevation when a space-occupying lesion occurs or the volume of brain parenchyma increases include a reduction in intracranial cerebrospinal fluid volume and intracranial blood volume. Intracranial compliance is reduced and ICP increases rapidly after compensatory mechanisms are exhausted. From: Chesnut[2]

herniation" (Table 2.2).[4] Brain shifting itself can lead to a reduced level of consciousness, but also produces characteristic signs of brain stem and motor pathway dysfunction, including an unreactive "blown" pupil, motor posturing, or autonomic dysfunction such as the Cushing reflex (hypertension and bradycardia).

Another major consequence of intracranial hypertension is a decrease in cerebral perfusion pressure (CPP), which can lead to global brain ischemia, which also contributes to decreased level of consciousness. CPP is calculated

Table 2.1 Common causes of intracranial hypertension

Infection	• Meningitis and encephalitis
	• Brain abscess
	• Subdural empyema
Vascular causes	• Acute ischemic stroke
	• Intracerebral hemorrhage
	• Subarachnoid hemorrhage
	• Cerebral venous sinus thrombosis
Tumors	• Primary brain tumor
	• Metastatic brain tumor
Traumatic brain injury	• Epidural hematoma
	• Subdural hematoma
	• Cerebral contusion
	• Diffuse axonal injury
Hydrocephalus	• Obstructive hydrocephalus
	• Communicating hydrocephalus
Miscellaneous	• Hypoxic-Ischemic encephalopathy
	• Acute fulminant liver failure
	• Severe hyponatremia
	• Posterior reversible encephalopathy syndrome
	• Post-carotid endarterectomy hyperperfusion syndrome
	• High-altitude cerebral edema

Source: Cadena et al.[12]

as mean arterial pressure (MAP) minus ICP. As CPP falls, cerebral blood flow (CBF) can fall to critical levels. This problem can be further exacerbated by failure of normal mechanisms of cerebral autoregulation. Cerebral perfusion in the late stages of herniation and ICP crisis can be further compromised by direct vascular compression against the falx or tentorium, resulting in secondary territorial infarcts of the anterior or posterior cerebral artery.

Table 2.2 Herniation syndromes

Herniation syndromes	Mechanisms	Signs and symptoms
Uncal herniation	Displacement of the medial part of the temporal lobe (uncus) to compress • Ipsilateral oculomotor nerve • Cerebral peduncle (ipsilateral or contralateral) • Reticular activating system in the midbrain • Posterior cerebral artery	• Ipsilateral pupillary dilation with impaired pupillary light reflex • Contralateral hemiparesis or motor posturing • Ipsilateral hemiparesis (Kernohan sign) • Stupor or coma • Ipsilateral infarction of occipital lobe
Central transtentorial herniation	Downward displacement of bilateral cerebral hemisphere to compress • Thalamus • Midbrain, pons, and medulla • Stretching of small penetrating vessels in the brain stem	• Stupor or coma • Bilateral decorticate or decerebrate posturing • Loss of upward eye movement (Parinaud syndrome) • Pupils in mid-position or small pupils • Rostral–caudal loss of brain stem reflexes • Brain stem infarction
Subfalcine herniation	Lateral displacement of the brain by a hemispheric mass lesion at the level of ventricles or above to compress • Contralateral cerebral hemisphere • Ipsilateral anterior cerebral artery	• Contralateral lower extremity paresis • May progress to bilateral motor posturing and coma • Ipsilateral infarction in the anterior cerebral artery area

Table 2.2 (cont.)

Herniation syndromes	Mechanisms	Signs and symptoms
Tonsillar herniation	Displacement of cerebellar tonsil into the foramen magnum to compress • Medulla • Fourth ventricle	• Stupor or coma from obstructive hydrocephalus • Quadriparesis • Neck stiffness • Apnea

From: Claassen et al.[4]

The effects of elevated ICP on CBF are complex and differ depending on whether intracranial compliance is normal or reduced.[5] Under normal circumstances, the cerebral arterioles have the ability to autoregulate and maintain CBF at a steady level by vasodilating when CPP is low, or vasoconstricting when CPP is elevated (Figure 2.2). When the system is compliant, increases in CBV that occur with low CPP (due to normal autoregulatory vasodilation) or high CPP (due to hydrostatic forces in the setting of perfusion pressure breakthrough) do not affect ICP. In states of reduced intracranial compliance, however, ICP increases at the extremes of CPP because increases in CBV can no longer be accommodated (Figure 2.2). For this reason, maintenance of CPP within an optimized and relatively narrow range (50–70 mmHg) is a central tenet of ICP management.

2.2.2 INTRACRANIAL PRESSURE WAVEFORM

The ICP waveform has three subcomponents (Figure 2.3). An initial percussion wave (P1) results from arterial pressure being transmitted from the choroid plexus. A second tidal wave (P2) is a reflection wave that is influenced by intracranial compliance, and the dicrotic wave (P3) is related to closure of the aortic valve. In normal circumstances, P1 is the tallest

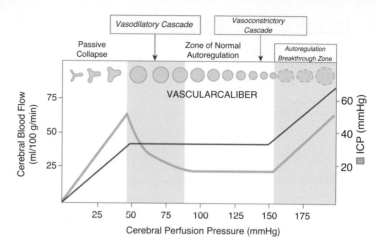

Figure 2.2 Relationship between extremes of cerebral perfusion pressure (CPP) and ICP in states of normal (black line) and reduced intracranial compliance (gray line). In the vasodilatory cascade zone, CPP reduction and intact pressure autoregulation lead to cerebral vasodilation and increased ICP; in this condition, ICP can be reduced by increasing mean arterial pressure (MAP) to raise CPP. In the autoregulation breakthrough zone, an increase in CPP leads to increased cerebral blood volume and ICP; in this condition, ICP can be further elevated when increasing MAP and CPP.
From: Rose and Mayer[24]

wave, followed by P2 and P3 (Figure 2.3A). When P2 is higher than P1, it suggests that intracranial compliance is reduced (Figure 2.3B).

2.2.3   PATHOLOGICAL PRESSURE WAVES

In patients with raised ICP, pathologic ICP waveforms may occur (Figure 2.3). Lundberg A waves (or plateau waves) represent prolonged periods of profoundly high ICP. They are ominous and abruptly occur when either CPP or intracranial compliance is low. Their duration ranges from minutes to hours, and their levels may reach as high as 50–100 mmHg. Plateau waves are characterized by "mirror" reductions in CPP (Figure 2.3C) and result from

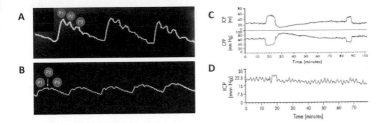

Figure 2.3 ICP waveforms. (A) normal intracranial waveforms consist of three subcomponents: P1 (percussion wave) results from arterial pressure being transmitted from choroid plexus; P2 (tidal wave) is a reflection wave that is influenced by intracranial compliance; and P3 (dicrotic wave) is related to closure of the aortic valve, with P1 being higher than P2 and P3. (B) ICP waveforms during reduced intracranial compliance (P2 is higher than P1). (C) Lundberg A waves (or plateau waves), which are intermittent periods (>10 minutes) of increasing ICP correlated with CPP reduction caused by cerebral vasodilatation during low CSF compensatory reserve. (D) Lundberg B waves represent shorter periods (<10 minutes) of intermittent ICP elevation without CPP reduction, indicating reduced intracranial compliance.
Reproduced from: Lele et al.[7] and Czosnyka and Pickard[8]

vasodilatory cascade physiology. As the brain senses that CPP and cerebral perfusion are too low, vasodilation occurs as part of normal autoregulation and drives ICP up. This further decreases CPP. The result is a vicious cycle: a state of maximal vasodilation, high ICP, and low CPP. Lundberg B waves are of shorter duration, with lower amplitude elevations (generally <20 mmHg and <10 minutes), that serve as a marker of reduced intracranial compliance (Figure 2.3D).

2.3 Intracranial Pressure Measurement

ICP monitoring is helpful for effective treatment. The diagnosis of increased ICP should not be made on clinical grounds alone. In order to diagnose increased ICP, it must be directly measured. Because of the invasive nature of ICP monitoring and the need for intensive care unit (ICU) management, patients should generally meet three criteria prior to placement of an ICP monitor:

(1) brain imaging reveals a space-occupying lesion or cisternal effacement, suggesting that the patient is at risk for high ICP;

(2) the patient is comatose (Glasgow Coma Scale [GCS] score of ≤8); and

(3) the prognosis is such that aggressive ICU treatment is indicated.

ICP value, trends, and waveforms should be interpreted together to assess intracranial compliance and for decision-making regarding treatment of ICP reduction. ICP monitoring also provides CPP values, which should be optimized within a target range using continuous infusion vasopressors or antihypertensive agents if necessary. Specific indications for ICP monitoring in patients with and without TBI are shown in Table 2.3.[3,6] The most common methods of ICP measurement are intraventricular and intraparenchymal ICP monitoring.

2.3.1 INTRAVENTRICULAR ICP MONITORING

Intraventricular ICP monitoring using an external ventricular drain (EVD) connected to a pressure transducer is considered the gold standard for measuring ICP.[2,7] The EVD should be zeroed to atmospheric pressure and leveled at the external auditory meatus using either a carpenter bubble or a laser level.[7] Intraventricular catheter placement may be difficult in patients with severe brain edema and compressed lateral ventricles. An EVD also allows for CSF drainage to reduce ICP and for treatment of hydrocephalus; drainage cannot be performed simultaneously with ICP measurement unless the catheter is equipped with a pressure microsensor at the tip. The CSF should not be drained faster than 20 ml/hour; overdrainage of CSF may result in bridging vein tears and subdural hematoma.[7]

Table 2.3 Indications for intracranial pressure monitoring

Traumatic brain injury	Nontraumatic brain injury
GCS ≤8 with abnormal head CT	• Patients with hydrocephalus or at high risk for developing hydrocephalus
• Intracranial hematoma	
• Cerebral contusion	• SAH, ICH, and other non-TBI conditions in patients who are at risk of elevated ICP based on clinical and/or imaging features
• Brain swelling	
• Brain herniation	
• Compressed basal cisterns	
GCS ≤8 with normal head CT and ≥2 of the following:	• All poor-grade SAH patients should be considered for multimodality monitoring
• Age >40 years	• Patients who undergo hemicraniectomy in the setting of cerebral edema
• Unilateral or bilateral motor posturing	
• Systolic blood pressure <90 mmHg	

From: Carney et al.[3] and Helbok et al.[6]

CT, computed tomography; GCS, Glasgow Coma Scale; ICH, intracranial hemorrhage; SAH, subarachnoid hemorrhage; TBI, traumatic brain injury

2.3.2 INTRAPARENCHYMAL ICP MONITORING

In this method, an intraparenchymal catheter with a pressure transducer is inserted through a skull bolt approximately 15 mm into the cranium.[1,8] The pressure transducer needs to be calibrated (so that atmospheric pressure is recognized as 0 mmHg) prior to insertion; it usually cannot be re-zeroed after placement. This technique allows for continuous ICP monitoring and can be used in the case of compressed and small lateral ventricles; however, it does not allow therapeutic CSF drainage. Other forms of multimodality neuromonitoring, such as brain tissue oxygen tension and cerebral microdialysis, can be placed together with the parenchymal ICP monitor using a multi-lumen bolt.

2.3.3 COMPLICATIONS

Complications of ICP monitoring include infection, intracranial hemorrhage, and catheter malfunction. The rate of meningitis and ventriculitis and intracranial bleeding is substantially higher with intraventricular catheters than with intraparenchymal monitors.[8] Coagulopathy should always be corrected before insertion of an ICP monitor. Strict sterile technique during insertion and manipulation of an EVD, along with early discontinuation, are the best defenses against ventriculostomy-related infection (VRI), which occurs in 5–15% of cases. VRI often leads to a need for extended drainage, treatment, and may worsen neurological outcome.

2.4 Intracranial Hypertension Management

The goals of intracranial hypertension management are to reduce ICP, prevent brain herniation, and maintain adequate CPP to ensure adequate CBF and prevent cerebral ischemia.[3,9,10] The specific cause of intracranial hypertension should be identified and treated as soon as possible. A stepwise algorithm for management of intracranial hypertension has been proposed for patients with severe TBI. This guidance can also be adapted for managing non-TBI patients who have elevated ICP. The algorithm consists of four tiers (Table 2.4), each containing a number of potential interventions that can be employed concurrently. It is not necessary to strictly follow every

Table 2.4 Stepwise algorithm for management of intracranial hypertension[10]

Tier zero: general measures to prevent further ICP elevation and secondary brain injury
- ICU admission
- Endotracheal intubation and mechanical ventilation (oxygen saturation target ≥94%)
- Serial neurological examination off sedation
- Head of bed elevation to 30–45° with the patient's head in the midline position
- Analgesia and sedation for pain control and to prevent agitation
- Maintenance of euvolemia with isotonic crystalloid (avoid hypotonic solutions)
- Seizure prophylaxis with levetiracetam for one week
- Fever control
- Maintain hemoglobin >7 g/dl
- Arterial catheter placement for cerebral perfusion pressure calculation
- Central venous catheterization
- End-tidal carbon dioxide monitoring

Tier one: initial treatment of intracranial hypertension
- Increase dose of analgesia and sedation to lower ICP
- Maintain $PaCO_2$ at low end of normal (35–38 mmHg)
- Intermittent bolus hyperosmolar therapy
- CSF drainage via external ventricular drain
- Maintain CPP between 60 and 70 mmHg or individualize CPP target based on multimodality monitoring data:
- ICP <20 mmHg
- $PbtO_2$ >20 mmHg
- The lowest pressure reactivity index (PR_x) or oxygen reactivity index (OR_x)
- Cerebral microdialysis: Lactate <4 mmol/l, lactate-to-pyruvate ratio (LPR) <25, glucose >0.8 mmol/l

Tier two: treatment of refractory intracranial hypertension
- Hyperventilation to target $PaCO_2$ of 25–35 mmHg (with $PbtO_2$ monitoring)
- A trial dose of NMBAs. Continuous infusion of these agents should be considered only if the ICP is reduced after the trial bolus dose

Table 2.4 (cont.)

- Perform MAP challenge to assess cerebral static pressure autoregulation status and to individualize MAP and CPP target

Tier three: treatment of superrefractory intracranial hypertension
- Secondary decompressive craniectomy
- Mild hypothermia (35–36 °C)
- Barbiturate coma

From: Hawryluk et al.[10]

ICP, intracranial pressure; $PaCO_2$, arterial partial pressure of carbon dioxide; mmHg, millimeter of mercury; CSF, cerebrospinal fluid; MAP, mean arterial pressure; NMBAs, neuromuscular blocking agents

step within each tier. Management should be individualized based on clinical judgment depending on the disease process and the patient's clinical trajectory. Neurosurgical intervention (craniotomy, ventricular drainage, or both) should always be considered the first-line treatment for patients with acute life-threatening ICP from trauma, subarachnoid, or intracerebral hemorrhage. In this setting, the tiered algorithm is intended to guide postoperative management in the ICU. Corticosteroids can be given in case of cerebral edema associated with brain tumor or brain abscess, but it is not recommended for treatment of cerebral edema from other causes.

2.4.1 TIER ZERO: BASELINE MEASURES

This tier consists of uniform general measures to prevent ICP elevation and can be applied for patients at risk for intracranial hypertension regardless of the ICP value. Such patients should be admitted to an ICU. Comatose patients should receive endotracheal intubation and mechanical ventilation to prevent airway compromise and hypoxemia, with an oxygen saturation target ≥94%. The head of the bed should be elevated to 30–45° with the patient's head in the midline position to optimize venous return from the brain. Serial neurological examination during sedation interruptions should be performed on a regular basis to assess level of consciousness and detect neurological deterioration. Analgesia and sedation should initially be given in the lowest dose needed for pain control and to prevent agitation, but not in excess for ICP reduction. A commonly used combination is intravenous fentanyl 25–100 µg/hour and propofol 5–50 µg/kg/minute titrated to light sedation. Isotonic crystalloid should be given for maintenance of euvolemia. Hypotonic solutions should be avoided because free water tends to accumulate in injured brain tissue due to an increased local concentration of osmotically active molecules, worsening brain edema and ICP. Seizure prophylaxis with levetiracetam 750–1,500 mg twice daily or phenytoin 100 mg three times a day for one week reduces the risk of early seizures from approximately 14% to 4%.[11] Causes of fever should be identified and treated, and body temperature of ≥38 °C should be controlled. Red blood cell transfusion is standard of care if hemoglobin falls below 7 g/dl. Arterial catheterization is necessary for continuous blood pressure monitoring and CPP calculation. Central venous catheterization and end-tidal carbon dioxide ($ETCO_2$) monitoring should be considered.

2.4.2 TIER ONE: FIRST RESPONSE TO ICP CRISIS

Tier-one treatment should be initiated when intracranial hypertension is established. The dose of analgesia and sedation can be increased to lower ICP. Deeper sedation reduces patient-ventilator dyssynchrony and elevated intrathoracic and central venous pressures, translating into lower CBV and ICP. The arterial partial pressure of carbon dioxide ($PaCO_2$) should be maintained at low end of normal (35–38 mmHg). Intermittent boluses of hyperosmolar therapy, either mannitol or hypertonic saline (Table 2.5), can be administered to reduce brain water

Table 2.5 Bolus osmotherapy: mannitol versus hypertonic saline

	Mannitol	Hypertonic saline
Dose	20% mannitol 0.25–1 g/kg intravenously over 5–15 minutes, may be repeated as frequently as every 30 minutes as needed	23.4% NaCl 30 ml, or 7.5% NaCl 75 ml, or 5% NaCl 100 ml, or 3% NaCl 150 ml intravenously over 5–15 minutes, may be repeated as frequently as every 30 minutes as needed
Patient selection	Mannitol, an osmotic diuretic, is the agent of choice for patients with congestive heart failure, pulmonary edema, hypertension, or fluid overload	Hypertonic saline increases intravascular volume and arterial blood pressure, making it the agent of choice in the setting of hypotension or hypovolemia
Adverse effects	Volume depletion Hypotension Hypokalemia Metabolic alkalosis Acute kidney injury Hyperglycemia	Cardiogenic pulmonary edema Hypernatremia Hyperchloremic metabolic acidosis Osmotic demyelination syndrome

From: Ropper[13] and Chesnut et al.[20]

content and the volume of brain parenchyma.[12,13] Mannitol should not be used in patients who are hypovolemic and hypotensive, and hypertonic saline should not be used in patients with increased risk of cardiogenic pulmonary edema. Non-bolus continuous infusion of mannitol or 2% or 3% hypertonic saline with the goal of establishing and maintaining an elevated serum sodium goal is not recommended because they fail to create the acute osmotic gradients that result in water clearance from edematous brain tissue.[14] Similarly, scheduled infusions of hyperosmolar therapy or intravenous furosemide are not recommended when ICP is monitored.

Bolus osmotherapy should generally be used to reduce elevated ICP or brain tissue shifting resulting in neurological deterioration. CSF can be drained via an intraventricular catheter; placement of an EVD for CSF drainage may be necessary if an intraparenchymal catheter is used initially. Lumbar CSF drainage is not recommended as it can lead to brain herniation. CPP should be maintained between 60 and 70 mmHg or individualized based on multimodality monitoring data (see later) to prevent ischemia. Routinely increasing CPP >90 mmHg is not recommended without multimodality neuromonitoring. Electroencephalography (EEG) should be monitored to detect and treat electrographic seizures in comatose patients.

2.4.3 TIER TWO: NAVIGATING REFRACTORY ICP

Treatments in this tier can be considered when intracranial hypertension is refractory to tier-one measures. Hyperventilation to lower target $PaCO_2$ levels of 25–35 mmHg can be performed and may be very effective if cerebral vasodilation and increased CBV are important components of the patient's condition. Due to the concern for extreme hyperventilation resulting in excessive cerebral vasoconstriction and brain ischemia, concurrent monitoring of brain tissue oxygen tension ($PbtO_2$) is recommended to ensure that this does not occur. Neuromuscular blocking agents (NMBAs) can be tried, but continuous infusions of these agents should be considered only if a trial bolus dose is effective and other tier-two interventions are failing. Cisatracurium 0.1–0.2 mg/kg or rocuronium 0.6–1.2 mg/kg are commonly used NMBAs for ICP control.

A *CPP challenge* produced with a trial of norepinephrine (5–30 μg/min) can be considered to assess cerebral static pressure autoregulation status and to optimize the CPP target. If autoregulation is intact, the patient is hypotensive, and vasodilatory cascade physiology is present (Figure 2.2). An increase in CPP will result in cerebral vasoconstriction, leading to decreased cerebral blood volume and ICP. Care must be taken, however, because if autoregulation is impaired, an increase in CPP may drive perfusion pressure breakthrough and further increase ICP. Other treatments that affect ICP, including sedative drug dose adjustments, hyperosmolar therapy, and the amount of CSF drainage, should not be changed during this procedure. A MAP challenge should be performed under the supervision of an experienced physician, and the procedure should be stopped immediately if the patient has neurological deterioration or an increase in ICP.

2.4.4   TIER THREE: SALVAGE MEASURES FOR SUPERREFRACTORY ICP

Treatment options in tier three for superrefractory intracranial hypertension, defined as failure of multiple tier-one and two measures to control intracranial hypertension, consist of rescue decompressive craniectomy, mild hypothermia (35–36 °C) and barbiturate coma. These interventions are problematic in that all can lead to serious complications, and none have been shown to improve functional outcomes, making them last-ditch measures to prevent devastating neurological injury, "ICP checkmate," or progression to brain death.

Pentobarbital High-dose barbiturate therapy, given in doses equivalent to those inducing general anesthesia, can effectively lower ICP in patients refractory to tier-two measures.[15] The effect of pentobarbital is multifactorial but most likely stems from coupled decreases in cerebral metabolism, blood flow, and blood volume. Pentobarbital typically requires a loading dose of 5 to 20 mg/kg, given in repeated 5 mg/kg boluses, until a state of flaccid coma with preserved pupillary reactivity is attained. Pentobarbital can cause profound hypotension and usually requires the use of vasopressors to maintain CPP at or higher than 60 mmHg. Maintenance doses are usually 1 to 4 mg/kg/hr. Continuous EEG monitoring should be used, with the infusion rate titrated to ICP and a burst-suppression pattern with bursts every 2–10 seconds. The infusion can be discontinued abruptly, with a washout period lasting from 24 to 96 hours. Complications include hypotension; immunosuppression; a rare "metabolic infusion syndrome" characterized by lactic acidosis, vasodilatory shock, and renal failure; and severe critical illness neuromyopathy due to prolonged immobilization in the majority of patients.

Hypothermia Lowering body temperature to 33 °C can reduce ICP elevations that are refractory to CPP optimization, osmotherapy, and hyperventilation, as an alternative to pentobarbital anesthesia.[16] Hypothermia has risks and should not be used indiscriminately as a general neuroprotective measure; in the Eurotherm3235 trial cooling as a first-line intervention for ICP elevation resulted in increased mortality.[17] Advanced feedback-controlled technology to rapidly and precisely cool the patient, in the form of an adhesive surface cooling system or endovascular heat exchange catheter, is typically required. A stepwise anti-shivering protocol should be used, which escalates from buspirone, magnesium infusion, and skin-counter-warming, up to sedation with dexmedetomidine or fentanyl. After cooling, the patient can be gradually rewarmed to 37 °C at a rate of 0.20–0.33 °C/hr. Complications of hypothermia accumulate with longer duration of cooling and include shivering, immunosuppression, coagulopathy, cardiovascular depression, arrhythmias, hyperglycemia, ileus, and rebound hyperkalemia during rewarming.[16]

Decompressive Craniectomy The ultimate step to take when confronted with superrefractory ICP is to decompress the cranial vault. Decompression of the cranium allows the brain to swell out of the skull defect and is the definitive intervention for severe ICP. In the RESCUEicp trial, which randomized severe TBI patients who suffered ICP >25 mmHg for 12–25 hours despite tier-one and two interventions, craniectomy resulted in a significant mortality reduction (27% vs 49%) compared to continued medical therapy alone.[18] Use of craniectomy only as a salvage intervention appears to be important, however. In the DECRA trial, which randomized TBI patients to craniectomy versus continued medical (largely barbiturate) therapy at the first sign of ICP elevation, craniectomy resulted in *increased* disability with no effect on mortality.[19]

2.5 Multimodality Monitoring

A multicenter randomized-controlled trial conducted to evaluate the efficacy of ICP data-guided therapy of patients with severe TBI (GCS of ≤8) in South America (BEST-TRIP) was unable to demonstrate an improvement in survival rate or functional outcome between patients managed with and without ICP monitoring.[20] Since secondary brain injury can occur despite ICP being less than 20 mmHg, ICP control alone may not be sufficient to improve patient outcome. Multimodality monitoring (MMM) combines ICP/CPP monitoring with additional brain physiological and biochemical variables such as brain perfusion, oxygenation, metabolism, and electrical function. Early detection of secondary brain injury captured by MMM may prevent permanent neuronal damage if proper treatments are provided in time. Physiological data derived from MMM (i.e. brain oxygen tension, autoregulation index, or cerebral lactate/pyruvate ratio) can be used to individualize CPP targets and create an optimized physiological environment for the severely injured brain.[21]

2.5.1   BRAIN OXYGENATION MONITORING

Brain tissue oxygenation is an indicator of adequacy of cerebral oxygen delivery. In multiple observational studies, it has been demonstrated that brain tissue hypoxia in comatose patients is associated with poor outcome (e.g. disability or death at follow-up).[2,22] Parenchymal brain tissue oxygen tension ($PbtO_2$) is the most accurate method of brain oxygenation monitoring. The $PbtO_2$ probe samples 15 mm^3 of brain volume around the catheter tip. In this technique, a $PbtO_2$ catheter is inserted via a bolt into the white matter in parallel to the intraparenchymal ICP monitor. The catheter position must be confirmed by a brain CT scan. A 60-minute equilibration period is required after catheter placement, and an oxygen challenge with 100% fraction of inspired oxygen for 15 minutes should be performed daily before data interpretation: a threefold increase in $PbtO_2$ after oxygen challenge indicates proper catheter function. Normal value of $PbtO_2$ ranges from 23 to 35 mmHg. Brain tissue hypoxia is defined as $PbtO_2$ of <20 mmHg. Measures to treat brain tissue hypoxia by increasing oxygen delivery include intravascular volume optimization and CPP augmentation, ventilator adjustment to correct arterial hypoxemia or alkalosis-related vasoconstriction, or red blood cell transfusion to improve cerebral oxygen delivery in the setting of anemia. Measures to reduce oxygen consumptions include treatment of fever and seizures, and the use of analgosedation to treat shivering or autonomic storming. A clinical trial of ICP combined with $PbtO_2$-guided therapy in severe TBI patients is ongoing (BOOST-3, ClinicalTrials.gov Identifier: NCT03754114).

Jugular bulb venous oxygen saturation ($SjvO_2$) is less accurate than $PbtO_2$. At least 13% of the brain volume must be ischemic to increase the oxygen extraction fraction and reduce $SjvO_2$. Normal $SjvO_2$ ranges from 55% to75%. Value <55% indicates cerebral ischemia and value >75% suggests cerebral hyperemia; both are associated with worse outcome. Near-infrared spectroscopy (NIRS) is a noninvasive method of brain oxygen monitoring. Given limited data, NIRS value alone should not be used as a target of treatment. NIRS can be integrated with arterial pressure monitoring to assess cerebral autoregulation.

2.5.2 CEREBRAL AUTOREGULATION MONITORING

Cerebral autoregulation is the capability of cerebral vasculature to maintain relatively constant CBF to protect the brain from ischemia and hyperemia when CPP is at high or low extremes (Figure 2.2).[23,24] When CPP is below the lower limit or above the upper limit of autoregulation, CBF becomes directly proportional to CPP, and ischemia or hyperemia will occur. In patients with acute brain injury, cerebral autoregulation monitoring can determine whether autoregulation is preserved or disrupted, and can identify the upper and lower limit of intact autoregulation. In this way autoregulation monitoring can help individualize the CPP target for a given patient.

Assessment of autoregulation is performed by calculating a moving correlation coefficient created by spontaneous fluctuations in driving pressure (MAP or CPP) as an input function and cerebral perfusion or blood volume as an output function. These correlation coefficients are generally calculated over a 5-minute window. This method requires software that can automatically calculate and display the autoregulation index together with ICP and CPP in real time. Measures of cerebral perfusion include mean flow velocity (mFV) in the middle cerebral artery measured by transcranial Doppler, $PbtO_2$, and regional cerebral oxygen saturation (rSO_2) measured by NIRS.[23] Commonly used autoregulation indices include the pressure reactivity index (PRx, the correlation coefficient between ICP and MAP), mean flow velocity index (the correlation coefficient between mFV and MAP), brain tissue oxygen pressure reactivity index (OR_x, the correlation coefficient between $PbtO_2$ and CPP) and cerebral oximetry index (the correlation coefficient between rSO_2 and MAP).

When only continuous ICP monitoring is used autoregulation status can be assessed with PR_x, the most commonly used index. If autoregulation is intact, an increase in MAP will result in cerebral vasoconstriction, resulting in reduced CBV and ICP, which yields a negative correlation coefficient. By contrast, in the setting of autoregulatory failure, a reduction in MAP will lead to cerebral vasodilatation and an increase in CBV and ICP, producing a positive correlation coefficient. The threshold for defining impaired autoregulation is a PR_x higher than +0.3. Optimal CPP (CPPopt) is defined as the CPP range that produces the lowest PR_x values, which should be negative (Figure 2.4).[25] The index is not perfect, in that PR_x clearly identifies a range of CPPopt in only 55% of monitored patients.

2.5.3 CEREBRAL METABOLISM MONITORING

Cerebral metabolism monitoring is a measurement of brain tissue biomarkers of cerebral ischemia and neuronal damage using cerebral microdialysis.[26] The common biomarkers include lactate, pyruvate, lactate-to-pyruvate ratio (LPR), glucose and glutamate. The microdialysis probe is a double-lumen flexible microcatheter covered by a semipermeable membrane; the probe can be inserted into brain parenchyma through a multi-lumen skull bolt in the same manner as a $PbtO_2$ catheter. The monitoring method is performed by infusing isotonic perfusate at a rate of 0.3 μL/min to allow diffusion of solutes from the interstitial fluid into the catheter lumen through the semipermeable membrane. Then the perfusate will move out of the brain via the other lumen and be collected hourly for biomarker analysis. Cerebral lactate >4 mmol/l, pyruvate <70 μmol/l and LPR >25 suggest cerebral ischemia. An increase in LPR with normal or high pyruvate indicates mitochondrial dysfunction, especially if $PbtO_2$ is >20 mmHg. Cerebral hypoglycemia is defined as brain glucose of <0.8 mmol/l, with normal levels in the range of 2.0 mmol/l. If cerebral hypoglycemia occurs together with increased LPR, it suggests cerebral ischemia.

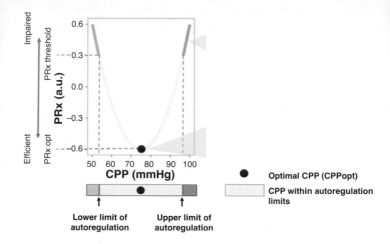

Figure 2.4 Relationships between cerebral perfusion pressure (CPP) and pressure reactivity index (PR$_x$). PR$_x$ is a moving correlation coefficient between mean arterial pressure (MAP) and intracranial pressure (ICP) calculated over a 5-minute window. If autoregulation is efficient, an increase in MAP will result in cerebral vasoconstriction and constant or decreased cerebral blood flow (CBF). Thus ICP will be unchanged or decreased. In contrast, a reduction in MAP will lead to cerebral vasodilatation, constant or increased CBF, and unchanged or increased ICP. Therefore, the PR$_x$ will be near zero or negative. If autoregulation is impaired, an increase or decrease in MAP will result in an increase or decrease in CBF and ICP, respectively. Hence the PR$_x$ will be a positive value approaching 1, suggesting a pressure passive condition. Very high or low CPP is correlated with high PR$_x$. Generally, PR$_x$ >0.3 indicates impaired autoregulation. The relationship between CPP and PR$_x$ can be approximated by fitting a U-shaped curve. The optimal CPP is the CPP correlating with the lowest PR$_x$ (PR$_x$ opt, black dot). The CPP values correlating with PR$_x$ of 0.3 indicate lower and upper limits of autoregulation.
From: Donnelly et al.[25]

2.6 Removal of ICP Monitoring

If an ICP monitor is placed in patients at risk of intracranial hypertension, but the ICP value is not elevated for at least 72 hours, the monitor can be removed.[2] If intracranial hypertension is established, removal of the ICP monitored can be considered once ICP is normal for at least 24 hours without ICP reduction therapy. Patient symptoms, brain imaging, and MMM data also influence a decision for removal of ICP monitor.

2.7 Conclusions

Intracranial hypertension is a life-threatening condition that if left unchecked can lead to brain herniation, cerebral ischemia, and brain death. Invasive ICP monitoring is often helpful for proper management, and the monitor should be inserted in comatose patients at high risk for elevated ICP. ICP values, trends, and waveforms should be used together to guide therapeutic decision-making. Patients with elevated ICP can be managed using a tiered stepwise strategy and depending on the etiology and severity of the insult. Multimodality neuromonitoring-guided therapy is a promising strategy that can early detect secondary brain injury, allow for individualized treatment targets, and provide improved situational awareness.

References

1. Czosnyka M, Pickard JD, Steiner LA. Principles of intracranial pressure monitoring and treatment. Handb Clin Neurol. 2017;140:67–89.
2. Chesnut RM. Intracranial pressure. In: Le Roux PD, Levine JM, Kofke WA, eds. Monitoring in neurocritical care. Philadelphia: Elsevier; 2013.
3. Carney N, Totten AM, O'Reilly C, Ullman JS, Hawryluk GW, Bell MJ, et al. Guidelines for the management of severe traumatic brain injury, 4th ed. Neurosurgery. 2017;80 (1):6–15.
4. Claassen J, Mayer SA, Brust JCM. Stupor and coma. In: Louis ED, Mayer SA, Rowland LP, eds. Merritt's *neurology*, 13th ed. Philadelphia: Wolters Kluwer; 2016, 153–63.
5. Donnelly J, Budohoski KP, Smielewski P, Czosnyka M. Regulation of the cerebral circulation: bedside assessment and clinical implications. Crit Care. 2016;20(1):129.

6. Helbok R, Olson DM, Le Roux PD, Vespa P. Intracranial pressure and cerebral perfusion pressure monitoring in non-TBI patients: special considerations. Neurocrit Care. 2014;21(Suppl 2):S85–94.

7. Lele AV, Hoefnagel AL, Schloemerkemper N, Wyler DA, Chaikittisilpa N, Vavilala MS, et al. Perioperative management of adult patients with external ventricular and lumbar drains: guidelines from the Society for Neuroscience in Anesthesiology and Critical Care. J Neurosurg Anesthesiol. 2017;29(3):191–210.

8. Marcus HJ, Wilson MH. Insertion of an intracranial-pressure monitor. N Engl J Med. 2015;373:e25.

9. Czosnyka M, Pickard JD. Monitoring and interpretation of intracranial pressure. J Neurol Neurosurg Psychiatry. 2004;75(6):813–21.

10. Hawryluk GWJ, Aguilera S, Buki A, Bulger E, Citerio G, Cooper DJ, et al. A management algorithm for patients with intracranial pressure monitoring: the Seattle International Severe Traumatic Brain Injury Consensus Conference (SIBICC). Intensive Care Med. 2019;45(12):1783–94.

11. Temkin NR, Dikmen SS, Wilensky AJ, Keihm J, Chabal S, Winn HR. A randomized, double-blind study of phenytoin for the prevention of post-traumatic seizures. N Engl J Med. 1990;323(8):497–502.

12. Cadena R, Shoykhet M, Ratcliff JJ. Emergency neurological life support: intracranial hypertension and herniation. Neurocrit Care. 2017;27(Suppl 1):82–88.

13. Ropper AH. Hyperosmolar therapy for raised intracranial pressure. N Engl J Med. 2012;367(8):746–52.

14. Cook AM, Morgan Jones G, Hawryluk GW, Mailloux P, McLaughlin D, Papangelou A, Samuel S, Tokumaru S, Venkatasubramanian C, Zacko C, Zimmermann LL. Guidelines for the acute treatment of cerebral edema in neurocritical care patients. Neurocrit Care. 2020;32:647–66.

15. Eisenberg HM, Frankowski RF, Contant CF, Marshall LF, Walker MD. High-dose barbiturate control of elevated intracranial pressure in patients with severe head injury. J Neurosurg. 1988;69(1):15–23.

16. Polderman KH, Herold I. Therapeutic hypothermia and controlled normothermia in the intensive care unit: practical considerations, side effects, and cooling methods. Crit Care Med. 2009;37:1101–20.

17. Andrews PJ, Sinclair HL, Rodriguez A, Harris BA, Battison CG, Rhodes JK, Murray GD. Hypothermia for intracranial hypertension after traumatic brain injury. N Engl J Med. December 17, 2015;373(25):2403–12.

18. Hutchinson PJ, Kolias AG, Timofeev IS, Corteen EA, Czosnyka M, Timothy J, Anderson I, Bulters DO, Belli A, Eynon CA, Wadley J. Trial of decompressive

craniectomy for traumatic intracranial hypertension. N Engl J Med. September 22, 2016;375:1119–30.

19. Cooper DJ, Rosenfeld JV, Murray L, et al. Decompressive craniectomy in diffuse traumatic brain injury. N Engl J Med. 2011;364:1493–502.

20. Chesnut RM, Temkin N, Carney N, Dikmen S, Rondina C, Videtta W, et al. A trial of intracranial-pressure monitoring in traumatic brain injury. N Engl J Med. 2012;367 (26):2471–81.

21. Le Roux P, Menon DK, Citerio G, Vespa P, Bader MK, Brophy GM, et al. Consensus summary statement of the international multidisciplinary consensus conference on multimodality monitoring in neurocritical care: a statement for healthcare professionals from the Neurocritical Care Society and the European Society of Intensive Care Medicine. Intensive Care Med. 2014;40(9):1189–209.

22. Oddo M, Bosel J. Monitoring of brain and systemic oxygenation in neurocritical care patients. Neurocrit Care. 2014;21(Suppl 2):S103–20.

23. Rivera-Lara L, Zorrilla-Vaca A, Geocadin RG, Healy RJ, Ziai W, Mirski MA. Cerebral autoregulation-oriented therapy at the bedside: a comprehensive review. Anesthesiology. 2017;126(6):1187–99.

24. Rose JC, Mayer SA. Optimizing blood pressure in neurological emergencies. Neurocrit Care. 2004;1(3):287–99.

25. Donnelly J, Czosnyka M, Adams H, Robba C, Steiner LA, Cardim D, et al. Individualizing thresholds of cerebral perfusion pressure using estimated limits of autoregulation. Crit Care Med. 2017;45(9):1464–71.

26. Hutchinson PJ, Jalloh I, Helmy A, Carpenter KL, Rostami E, Bellander BM, et al. Consensus statement from the 2014 international microdialysis forum. Intensive Care Med. 2015;41(9):1517–28.

3

Disorders of Temperature Regulation

Ameeta Karmarkar and Andrew M Naidech

Abstract

As the first vital sign, temperature occupies a prominent place in the initial assessment of a patient and is of particular significance in an acutely ill patient in the neurocritical care unit. Its interpretation, measurement, and clinical significance can be confounded by the disruption of the normal thermoregulatory mechanisms of the central nervous system, as well as various pharmacotherapies. This chapter aims to provide the reader with an overview of the clinical approach to fever in the neurocritical care unit. This will encompass a discussion of the common causes of fever, including serotonin syndrome, neuroleptic malignant syndrome, malignant hyperthermia, and paroxysmal sympathetic hyperreactivity. Finally, we describe how temperature can be leveraged as an evidence-based therapeutic tool to help improve neurologic outcomes after cardiac arrest.

3.1 Introduction

Temperature is a crucial and readily measurable variable in states of health and disease. The optimum temperature for cellular function is 37 °C. Core temperature is affected by circadian rhythms, exercise, and menstrual cycles but is maintained within a variation of 0.2–0.5 °C by adjustments of skin vasomotor responses. Fever is a physiologic response to inflammatory mediators commonly provoked by infections. A joint task force from the American College of Critical Care Medicine and the Infectious Diseases Society of America defines fever as a body temperature of 38.3 °C (101 °F) or higher.[1] Hypothermia is defined as a core body temperature of less than 35.0 °C.

3.2 Why Is Temperature Important in the Neurocritical Care Unit?

Sydenham once referred to fever as *"Nature's engine which she brings into the field to remove her enemy."* Fever has a long evolutionary history and has been recognized as a protective adaptive mechanism that promotes microbial killing and enhances leukocyte function. In any intensive care setting, it is a valuable indicator and should prompt a workup for the most common causes, such as infections and venous thromboembolism. In patients with subarachnoid hemorrhage (SAH), fever can be an indicator of vasospasm. Up to 60% of patients with acute stroke have fever. Acute temperature lability may be associated with herniation syndromes. Paroxysmal sympathetic hyperactivity is commonly seen in patients with severe traumatic brain injury (TBI).

Under normal circumstances, brain temperature is tightly regulated largely due to the intact blood–brain and blood–cerebrospinal fluid barriers. Neurons, in particular cerebellar Purkinje cells, are extremely sensitive to heat stress. Fever can therefore have more sinister implications for the acutely injured brain. Secondary injury from fever can occur due to proinflammatory effects, increased blood–brain barrier permeability, increased free radical production, glutamate release, and resultant excitotoxicity, all of which can exacerbate cerebral edema. Fever can also significantly raise intracranial pressure (ICP) and lower seizure threshold. Meta-analyses have demonstrated that fever at onset and in the acute setting after ischemic brain injury, intracerebral hemorrhage, and cardiac arrest has a negative impact on morbidity and mortality. Severe acute elevations in body temperature can cause systemic adverse effects, including electrolyte abnormalities (e.g. hypo- and hyperkalemia, hypo- and hypernatremia, hypoglycemia, hypophosphatemia, hypomagnesemia, and hypocalcemia), rhabdomyolysis, acute liver failure, disseminated intravascular coagulation, and myocardial injury.

While being vigilant about the maintenance of normothermia in acute neurologic disease, therapeutic hypothermia may be utilized for its neuroprotective benefit, which will be discussed below.

3.3 Normal Thermoregulatory Mechanisms

While the hypothalamus and skin are identified as having the major role in thermal regulation, nearly every tissue of the body is involved in the process. The medial preoptic/anterior hypothalamic area (POA) is the primary thermosensitive area in the central nervous system. Warm sensitive (WS) neurons in the POA integrate afferent input and depending on the level of their activity, trigger heat loss (vasodilation, sweating) and inhibit heat gain (cutaneous vasoconstriction, thermogenesis). WS neurons tonically inhibit the dorsomedial nucleus of the hypothalamus (DMH) and the caudal periaqueductal gray matter (PAG). Both the DMH and PAG activate the Nucleus Raphe Pallidus (RPa). The RPa stimulates heat gain via descending sympathetic pathways. Additional pathways to the limbic system, lower brain stem, the reticular formation, and spinal cord are also involved in heat gain responses. These two opposing influences counterbalance at a temperature "set point" of 37 °C.[2]

3.4 Physiologic Fever and Mechanism of Action of Antipyretics

Under physiologic conditions, a fever is commonly triggered by infections. The organum vasculosum in the anterior hypothalamus lacks a blood–brain barrier, thus allowing stimulation by pyrogenic substances. Pyrogens may be exogenous (e.g. microorganisms) or endogenous (e.g. interleukin (IL)-1, IL-6, tumor necrosis factor (TNF)-α), which act directly or via cytokines. Stimulation of the organum vasculosum leads to increased production of prostanoids, including prostaglandin (PG)E$_2$, which results in slowing the firing rate of the WS neurons. The "set-point" in the hypothalamus shifts upward and results in an increase in body temperature. Hyperthermia, on the other hand, is regarded as an elevation of core body temperature above the normal diurnal range due to failure of normal thermoregulation (Figure 3.1).

The antipyretic activity of nonsteroidal anti-inflammatory drugs (NSAIDs) is due to inhibition of prostaglandin synthesis. Acetaminophen reduces fever induced by pyrogens in parallel with reduction in levels of a PG-like material in the cerebrospinal fluid.

3.5 Measurement of Body Temperature

The core temperature represents that of the internal organs, which may not be accurately represented by measurements from the skin or other orifices. When feasible, the pulmonary artery temperature is considered the gold standard for core temperature. Other internal sites at which core temperature has been measured include the esophagus, intestines, rectum, and bladder. Urinary temperature

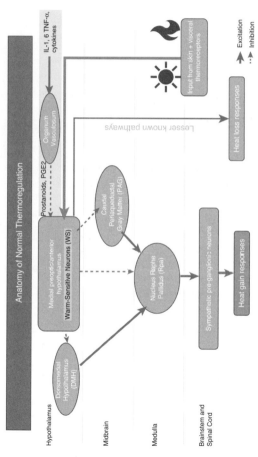

Figure 3.1 Anatomy of normal thermoregulation.

The warm-sensitive neurons (WS) in the medial preoptic/anterior hypothalamic area (POA) are the main integrators of thermal information. Afferent input is received by the WS neurons from heat sensitive receptors in the skin (via the spinothalamic tracts) and the viscera. Increased body temperature stimulates WS neuron activity. The nucleus raphe pallidus (RPa) plays a key role as its descending projections activate sympathetic preganglionic neurons, which trigger heat gain responses (skin vasoconstriction and nonshivering thermogenesis). The dorsomedial nucleus of the hypothalamus (DMH) and caudal periaqueductal gray (PAG) stimulate the RPa. WS neurons tonically inhibit the DMH, caudal periaqueductal PAG, and RPa, thus inhibiting heat gain. Through less elucidated descending pathways, the WS neurons also stimulate heat loss (vasodilation, sweating).

The area shaded in yellow in the top-right corner represents the pathogenesis of fever. Systemic inflammatory mediators stimulate the organum vasculosum in the anterior hypothalamus. The resultant synthesis of prostaglandin $(PG)E_2$ inhibits WS neuron activity thus resulting in a rise in body temperature or fever.

sensors require the presence of an indwelling catheter and a urine output of at least 10 ml/h. Rectal thermometry has essentially evolved into the standard for measuring core temperature, but does lag behind true visceral temperature fluctuations and may carry a small risk of trauma and infection. Oral temperature affords easier access, but is confounded by probe placement and exposure to ingested material and air. Furthermore, oral, bladder, and rectal temperatures are generally lower than brain temperatures, and this gradient is larger during fever.

3.6 Clinical Approach to Fever in the Neurocritical Care Unit

Fever in a critically ill patient can have a varied differential diagnosis depending on associated signs and symptoms, immunosuppression, the degree of elevation in temperature and relation to the length of stay (LOS) (Table 3.1).

It is commonly observed that most noninfectious fevers do not exceed 102 °F. However, in certain populations, infections may present with relative normothermia or even hypothermia. This includes the elderly, patients with open abdominal wounds, end-stage liver disease, heart failure, and burns, and patients receiving extracorporeal membrane oxygenation or continuous renal replacement therapy. In neutropenic patients, fever is defined as a single oral temperature of ≥38.3 °C (101 °F) or a temperature of ≥38.0 °C (100.4 °F) sustained over a 1-h period.

In our intensive care unit, the typical threshold to initiate an infectious workup is a core body temperature >101.5 °F (or 38.5 °C) in immunocompetent patients not presenting with other convincing signs of

Table 3.1 Fever in the neurocritical care unit: differential diagnosis and workup

Fever >101.5 °F Infectious

Differential diagnosis:	Associated Features	Workup
Pneumonia, particularly ventilator-associated pneumonia (VAP)	Increasing oxygen requirement, focal infiltrates, increased volume, purulence of secretions	Complete blood count, comprehensive metabolic panel, lactic acid, hepatic function panel including direct and indirect bilirubin
Central venous catheters (CVCs) (i.e. intravenous [IV] line infections)	Higher risk: TPN, immunosuppression, higher in femoral and internal jugular, nontunneled, bare as compared to antibiotic impregnated, multiple lumen, duration of insertion >1 week, repeated insertion	Blood cultures × 2 (repeat q48 h for persistent fevers) Nonbronchoscopic (or bronchoscopic, if indicated for mucus plugging, lobar collapse) bronchoalveolar lavage:
Clostridium difficile colitis	>3 loose bowel movements over 24 h, no laxatives for 48 h prior, abdominal distention, leukocytosis >20	Cell count, Gram stain and culture, respiratory viral panel, procalcitonin, MRSA PCR
Meningitis/Encephalitis	Existing intracranial shunts, external ventricular catheter, drains	Urinalysis and urine culture
Urosepsis	Indwelling urinary catheters	Cerebrospinal fluid from shunt/EVD/lumbar puncture
Intraabdominal sepsis	Recent abdominal procedures such as feeding tube placement, purulent discharge, abdominal guarding	Clostridium difficile stool PCR
	Patients with cirrhosis decompensated by ascites may be at risk for spontaneous bacterial peritonitis	Echocardiogram (transthoracic, transesophageal) if bacteremia or signs of septic embolization present
	Noncalculous cholecystitis in critically ill patients	

Differential Diagnoses	Associated Features	Workup
Wound infection Pressure-sore related infections	Chronically ill, bedbound patients, spinal cord injury	Right upper quadrant ultrasound if cholestatic jaundice, signs of cholestasis Examine skin for pressure sores, needle aspiration or deep tissue biopsy if purulent discharge, consider debridement/Plastic Surgery consult MRI if concern for underlying osteomyelitis Examination of all recent surgical sites Consider CT chest abdomen pelvis to look for loculated source of infection/abscess if no improvement, persistent bacteremia despite directed antibiotic therapy, and/or recent surgical intervention

Fever >101.5 °F Noninfectious

Differential Diagnoses	Associated Features	Workup
Acute thromboembolism		Low threshold to obtain bilateral lower extremity Dopplers CT-PE if clinically indicated
Transfusion associated fever	Recent blood product administration	Initiate protocol for suspected transfusion reaction if other signs present

Table 3.1 (cont.)

Fever >101.5 °F Noninfectious

Differential Diagnoses	Associated Features	Workup
Drug fever	Associated with beta-lactams, phenytoin, carbamazepine, phenobarbital	Include differential to look for eosinophilia and transaminitis, examine for rashes, consider Infectious Diseases consultation
Central fever	Typical onset within 72 h of admission	Diagnosis of exclusion
	More common in SAH, significant intraventricular hemorrhage, intracranial tumors	May be associated with paroxysmal sympathetic hyperthermia (PSH)
	Often persistent (>6 h for >2 consecutive days)	
Myocardial infarction		
Fat embolism		
Pancreatitis		
Benign postoperative fever		
Medication-associated syndromes (see Tables 3.2, 3.3)		
Malignancy		
Endocrine (thyrotoxcicosis, pheochromocytoma)		

infection. In patients with conditions such as acute stroke, traumatic brain injury, and recent cardiac arrest, efforts are usually made to maintain normothermia, but the provider should consider discontinuing antipyretics if evaluating for a true fever spike.

3.7 Neurologic Disorders and Temperature Regulation

A variety of disorders as well as commonly used medications can affect different levels of the normal thermoregulatory apparatus of the nervous system.

- *Afferent input:* Peripheral neuropathies and myelopathies can cause impaired cold perception as well as inappropriate cutaneous vasodilatation.
- *Central control:* Severe TBI, structural lesions of the brain stem and hypothalamus due to stroke or demyelination, limbic encephalitis, large hemispheric strokes, subarachnoid hemorrhage and raised intracranial pressure, particularly in the setting of acute hydrocephalus, can impact central temperature regulation. This may manifest as central fevers, paroxysmal sympathetic hyperreactivity (PSH), paroxysmal hypothermia, and/or temperature lability. Wernicke's encephalopathy and thalamic demyelination in multiple sclerosis may impair the generation of a thermoregulatory response in the hypothalamus. Hypopituitarism and myxedema can cause impaired thermoregulation commonly causing hypothermia. Agenesis of the corpus callosum can be associated with paroxysmal hyper- or hypothermia. Any condition that results in a depressed state of consciousness increases the risk of hypothermia, examples including dementia, post-ictal states, alcohol, or sedative drugs.

- *Efferent response:* The capacity to generate heat by muscle contraction as well as seek warmth quickly in a cold environment can be affected by several conditions that impair mobility, such as Parkinson's disease, stroke, spinal cord injury, or myopathy. Conversely, various medical conditions can impair heat-dissipating mechanisms or increase generation of body heat, leading to increased risk of hyperthermia. Multiple system atrophy, pure autonomic failure, and spinal cord transection impair thermoregulatory sweating. Heat generation from the sustained muscle contractions in status epilepticus may contribute to hyperthermia.

Other systemic disorders, including endocrine disorders such as hypothyroidism, hypoglycemia, and adrenal insufficiency, impair metabolic thermogenesis. Conditions such as thyrotoxicosis and pheochromocytoma may cause hyperthermia.

3.8 Anesthesia and Temperature Regulation

Thermoregulation during anesthesia – general or regional – is often significantly impaired by a number of mechanisms. The incidence of perioperative hypothermia is reported to be as high as 70% and is of major concern, particularly in lengthy procedures, and can predispose to complications such as poor wound healing, infections and coagulopathy. General anesthesia significantly alters thermoregulatory threshold, which is reduced from 37 °C to 34.5 °C. The interthreshold range is widened to ±4 °C, sweating threshold slightly elevated, and vasoconstriction threshold markedly lowered. Impairment of vasoconstriction responses affects redistribution of body heat. Shivering thermogenesis is impaired by all general anesthetics, even without muscle blockade.

3.9 Hyperthermia Associated with Medication Use (Table 3.2)

3.9.1 SEROTONIN SYNDROME

Serotonin syndrome is characterized by hyperthermia, agitation, tremor, myoclonus, muscle rigidity, hyperreflexia, and hyperhidrosis. Patients at risk include those taking multiple serotonin-selective reuptake inhibitors (SSRIs) or in combination with other drugs, such as meperidine, fentanyl, or tramadol, which enhance central serotonin availability. SSRIs can contribute to its development up to several weeks after discontinuation. Management includes supportive care, discontinuation of serotonergic agents, and sedation with benzodiazepines. Control of hyperthermia is critical. Patients with temperatures >41.1 °C require immediate sedation, frequently with neuromuscular blockade. Succinylcholine should be avoided if hyperkalemia is present. Hypertension and tachycardia can be managed with short acting agents such as esmolol or nitroprusside. Cyproheptadine is a histamine-1 receptor antagonist with nonspecific 5-HT1A and 5-HT2A antagonistic properties may be used if benzodiazepines and supportive care fail.

3.9.1.1 Hunter Serotonin Toxicity Criteria[3]

The criteria require the presence of *one* of the following classical features or groups of features:
- spontaneous clonus
- inducible clonus with agitation or diaphoresis
- ocular clonus with agitation or diaphoresis
- tremor and hyperreflexia
- hypertonia, temperature above 100.4 °F (38 °C), and ocular or inducible clonus

Table 3.2 Medications associated with hypothermia and hyperthermia

Medications	
Hypothermia	**Mechanism of Action**
Opiates	CNS depression, central mu and kappa receptor agonist
Barbiturates	CNS depression, impaired central thermoregulation
Benzodiazepines	CNS depression, impaired central thermoregulation
Bromocriptine	D2 receptor agonist in hypothalamus
Anesthesia	Multiple mechanisms (see section 3.7)
Alcohol intoxication	CNS depression, impaired thermoregulation
Neuromuscular blockade	Impaired shivering
Atypical antipsychotics (risperidone, clozapine, olanzapine, aripiprazole, quetiapine)	Alpha-adrenergic receptor antagonist, impaired peripheral heat gain mechanisms, central antagonism of the 5-HT-2-receptor
Hyperthermia	
Salicylates	Uncouple oxidative phosphorylation
Stimulant Drugs of Abuse	Increased synaptic norepinephrine, dopamine, and serotonin
Cocaine	Direct agonist at α1 and β adrenoreceptors in hypothalamus
Amphetamines	
Methamphetamines	

4-methylenedioxy-methamphetamine (MDMA or "ecstasy")	Peripheral mechanisms-activation of astrocytes and microglia, peripheral catecholamine release, increased skeletal muscle metabolism, peripheral vasoconstriction, cytokine formation and release
Anticholinergics	Impaired sweating
Dopamine antagonists	D2 receptor blockade in hypothalamus
Meperidine	Inhibition of shivering
Serotonergic drugs (SSRIs, MAOIs)	5 HT2 receptor agonism in hypothalamus
Carbonic anhydrase inhibitors (topiramate, acetazolamide, zonisamide)	Inhibit sweat production at level of glands

3.9.2   NEUROLEPTIC MALIGNANT SYNDROME (NMS)

Neuroleptic malignant syndrome is a potentially fatal, idiosyncratic condition that occurs in 0.2% of patients taking dopamine 2 receptor antagonists (see Table 3.3). Clinical signs consist of hyperthermia, diffuse "lead pipe" rigidity, hyperhidrosis, tachycardia, labile blood pressure, tremor, dysarthria, and delirium. Laboratory findings typically include elevations in creatine kinase, liver enzymes, and white blood count combined with low serum iron. Central dopaminergic impairment with defective heat dissipation has been proposed to explain the hyperthermia.

Treatment for NMS includes removal of all dopamine blocking agents as well as other contributors such as serotonergic drugs, anticholinergics, and lithium. Benzodiazepines, supportive care, and management of associated organ dysfunction constitute the main approach. Dantrolene is a direct-acting skeletal muscle relaxant and reduces skeletal heat production and rigidity. It does carry a risk of hepatotoxicity. Bromocriptine, a dopamine agonist, can be continued for 10 days after NMS is controlled and then tapered. Amantadine has dopaminergic and anticholinergic effects and is another alternative. Other less commonly used options include apomorphine, carbamazepine, and bupropion. Most episodes resolve within 2 weeks, but cases persisting for up to 6 months with residual catatonia and motor signs have been reported. Electroconvulsive therapy (ECT) may be considered in patients not responding to other treatments or in whom nonpharmacologic psychotropic treatment is needed.

3.9.3   MALIGNANT HYPERTHERMIA

Malignant hyperthermia is an autosomal-dominant inherited disorder of skeletal muscle calcium regulation that in up to 70% of cases is associated

Table 3.3 A comparison of serotonin syndrome, neuroleptic malignant syndrome, anticholinergic toxicity, and malignant hyperthermia

	Serotonin Syndrome (SS)	Neuroleptic Malignant Syndrome (NMS)	Anticholinergic Toxicity	Malignant Hyperthermia (MH)
Medications commonly implicated	Antidepressants: Selective serotonin reuptake inhibitors (SSRIs) Serotonin-norepinephrine reuptake inhibitors (SNRIs) Tricyclic antidepressants (TCAs) Monoamine oxidase inhibitors (MAOIs) Lithium Antimicrobials: Linezolid, Fluconazole, Ciprofloxacin Antiemetics: Ondansetron, Metoclopramide Opioids: meperidine, fentanyl, tramadol Antiepileptics: valproate, carbamazepine Drugs of abuse: cocaine, MDMA (ecstasy), amphetamines	Antipsychotics_D2 receptor antagonists_ Antiemetics: Metoclopramide, promethazine, prochlorperazine Withdrawal of dopaminergic agents in parkinsonism	Antihistamines (diphenhydramine) Tricyclic antidepressants (TCAs) Antiemetics (Scopolamine) Mydriatics (Atropine, Cyclopentolate) Parkinsonism medications (Benztropine, Trihexyphenidyl) Bronchodilators (Ipratropium) Antipsychotics (chlorpromazine, fluphenazine, thioridazine) Bladder antispasmodics (oxybutynin, tolterodine)	Inhaled anesthetic (halothane, isoflurane, enflurane) +/− succinylcholine Predisposing factor: Mutations encoding for RYR1 (ryanodine receptos) or DHP (didhydropyridine) receptor

Table 3.3 (cont.)

	Serotonin Syndrome (SS)	Neuroleptic Malignant Syndrome (NMS)	Anticholinergic Toxicity	Malignant Hyperthermia (MH)
Onset	Within 24 h	Typically days to <2 weeks of exposure	<2 h	<1 h
Time course	24 h	Days to weeks	Hours to days	First sign is rise in ETCO2 Hours
Common features	Hyperthermia Tachycardia Altered mental status (agitation more severe in NMS)			
Distinguishing clinical features	Myoclonus, including ocular clonus Ataxia **Hyperreflexia** Mydriasis Shivering **Diarrhea Nausea, vomiting**	**Severe Lead pipe rigidity** Bradyreflexia **Agitation**	Flushing, mydriasis, loss of accommodation, **anhidrosis, urinary retention, constipation** **Lilliputian hallucinations** Seizures	Generalized rigidity especially **masseter** **Rapid rise in end tidal CO2** and temperature
Common Laboratory Abnormalities 5	Elevated **CK (highest in NMS, >1000)**, WBC, LDH, transaminitis, myoglobinuric renal failure, metabolic acidosis, shock, DIC			
Distinguishing Features	Specific with TCA toxicity: EKG abnormalities: prolonged QT, QRS	low serum iron CK elevations more pronounced		Mixed metabolic and **respiratory acidosis** Acute hyperkalemia (peaked T waves, ventricular arrythmias)

| Treatment in addition to supportive care and discontinuation of agent(s) | Benzodiazepines
Cyproheptadine 12 mg PO followed by 2 mg q12 h | Benzodiazepines
Dantrolene 1–2.5 mg/kg IV
Bromocriptine 2.5 mg q6-8 h
Amantadine 100 mg PO q12 h | Physostigmine (not in TCA poisoning) 0.5–2 mg IV q10-30 min
Benzodiazepines
Na bicarbonate if prolonged QRS | Stop anesthetic, increase fresh gas flow to enhance elimination
Dantrolene loading dose 2.5 mg/kg IV, additional 1 mg/kg IV as needed
Avoid calcium channel blocker use with dantrolene |

with mutations of the RYR1 gene encoding ryanodine receptor type 1. Approximately 1% result from mutations of CACNA1S, which encodes a skeletal muscle calcium channel. Upon exposure to volatile anesthetic agents, either alone or in combination with a depolarizing muscle relaxant, genetically predisposed individuals develop uncontrolled skeletal muscle hypermetabolism causing hyperthermia, muscle rigidity, tachycardia, acidosis, and hyperkalemia. Rhabdomyolysis with subsequent elevation in creatine kinase may lead to renal failure. An early unexplained rise in end tidal carbon dioxide levels despite adequate ventilation can be the first indicator of its development, along with diffuse muscle rigidity, particularly involving the masseters. Prompt administration of dantrolene is crucial, along with other supportive management.

3.10 Paroxysmal Sympathetic Hyperactivity (PSH)

Excessive sympathetic nervous system activity can develop after severe acquired brain injury, and its recognition has been historically hindered by lack of consistent definitions. An international expert consensus group in 2014 established a definition as follows: "A syndrome, recognized in a subgroup of survivors of severe acquired brain injury, of simultaneous, paroxysmal transient increases in sympathetic (elevated heart rate, blood pressure, respiratory rate, temperature, sweating) and motor (posturing) activity."[4]

A review of 349 PSH case reports found that about 80% followed TBI, 10% followed anoxic brain injury, 5% followed stroke, and the remaining 5% occurred in association with hydrocephalus, tumors, hypoglycemia, infections, or unspecified causes. In patients with TBI, PSH has been associated with diffuse axonal injury, younger age, and a greater burden of focal parenchymal lesions on CT. Patients with midbrain and pontine lesions are at increased risk of developing PSH, as are those with lesions in the periventricular white matter, corpus callosum, and deep gray nuclei. PSH has been described in patients at all stages following brain injury – from early critical care through to the rehabilitation phase, but may be masked by sedative use during the early course. Opioids, particularly morphine, may be helpful in modulating the allodynic responses as well as central pathways. Other sedatives, such as midazolam, have also been used. Propranolol, a nonselective β-blocker, crosses the blood-brain barrier owing to its lipophilicity, and its use has been shown to be independently associated with lower mortality when compared with other β-blockers. The α2-adrenergic drugs (clonidine, dexmedetomidine) act through central and peripheral adrenergic inhibition but may be less effective in controlling body temperature.

Other modulators of sympathetic paroxysms include bromocriptine (especially for temperature control and sweating), gabapentin, baclofen, and dantrolene. Table 3.4 summarizes some of the commonly used medications for treating PSH. Of equal importance is supportive therapy, such as physical therapy, positioning, temperature management, and nutrition, because of significant increases in energy expenditure associated with paroxysms.[5]

3.11 Therapeutic Temperature Management (TTM) in Neurocritical Care

"Extreme remedies are very appropriate for extreme diseases." — Hippocrates

The idea that hypothermia can be neuroprotective originated in antiquity, based on observations that infants abandoned and exposed to cold often

Table 3.4 Treatment of paroxysmal sympathetic hyperreactivity (PSH)

Medication	Dosing	Features of PSH affected	Major adverse effects
Opioids (morphine, fentanyl)	Morphine 1–10 mg IV q1–2 h Fentanyl 25–100 mcg IV q1–2 h or patch	Nearly all features	Sedation, respiratory depression, constipation, tolerance
Beta-blockers (nonselective, lipophilic- propranolol)	Propranolol 20–60 mg PO q 4–6 h	Tachycardia, hypertension, diaphoresis	Hypotension, bradycardia
α2 agonists	Clonidine 100 μg PO q 8–12 h, max 1.2 mg/day Dexmedetomidine 0.2–1.2 μg/kg/h	Hypertension tachycardia	Hypotension, bradycardia, sedation, risk of withdrawal with long term use
Bromocriptine (Dopamine D2 receptor agonist)	1.25 mg PO q12 h, titrate to a maximum of 40 mg/day	Temperature	Confusion, agitation, dyskinesia, nausea, hypotension
Gabapentin	100 mg PO q 8 h, PO; max 4800 mg/day	Spasticity and allodynic responses	Mild sedation, weight gain
Baclofen (GABAb agonist in spinal cord)	5 mg q8 h, PO; max 80 mg/day	Spasticity, dystonia	Sedation, risk of withdrawal with long term use
Benzodiazepines	Lorazepam 1–4 mg IV, Midazolam 1– 10 mg IV, q1–2 h	Agitation, hypertension, tachycardia, posturing	Sedation, respiratory depression, tachyphylaxis, risk of withdrawal with long term use
Dantrolene	0.5–2 mg/kg IV q 6–12 h; max 10 mg/kg/day	Posturing and muscular spasms	Hepatotoxicity, respiratory depression

survived for prolonged periods. Clinical trials on hypothermia, usually very deep (30 °C or lower), were first started in the 1960s, but they were soon discontinued because of adverse effects and unclear benefits.

Animal studies that demonstrated a neuroprotective effect of mild hypothermia (32–35 °C) against cerebral ischemia and hypoxemia prompted a renewed clinical interest in hypothermia in the 1980s. Conversely, elevated temperature following cardiac arrest has been shown to be associated with unfavorable neurological outcome. For each degree rise in temperature above 37 °C there was an increased association with severe disability, coma, or persistent vegetative state. Hyperthermia increases neurotransmitter release and accelerates production of oxygen radicals during the reperfusion period, causing excitatory amino acid release and calcium shifts, which can in turn lead to mitochondrial damage and apoptosis. Targeted temperature management is thought to suppress many of these biochemical alterations associated with reperfusion injury.

In humans, the only condition in which therapeutic hypothermia has been shown to improve neurological outcomes is following cardiac arrest.

3.11.1   IMPLEMENTATION OF TTM

According to international guidelines, temperature should be maintained at 32 °–36 °C for at least 24 h following cardiac arrest, whereas rewarming should not increase more than 0.5 °C per h.

Targeted temperature management can be divided into three phases (Figure 3.2):

- intentional change from current temperature to lower temperature – "induction";
- maintenance of that temperature for a time – "maintenance"; and
- change to a new temperature value by increase in temperature at a specific rate to a normothermic target – "rewarming."

Implementation of Therapeutic Temperature Management (TTM) after Cardiac Arrest

INDUCTION

- Core temperature monitoring: Foley probe (preferred) or rectal if urine output < 10 ml/h
- Baseline neurologic exam
- Initiate cooling with target temperature 32–36 °C. Select specific goal
- Preferred technique is surface cooling pads with feedback control
- Set ventilator proximal airway temperature to <96.8°F (36 °C)
- Short acting sedation to prevent shivering (fentanyl), lorazepam, propofol
- Palpate mandible Q15 minutes to assess for shivering, treat accordingly (see Figure 1.3)

MAINTENANCE

- Monitor electrolytes (K, Mg, phos), lactate* Q4h, coagulation studies q12 hours
- Avoid hypovolemia, replete with isotonic fluids
- Surveillance blood cultures 12 h from start of cooling
- Consider continuous EEG monitoring and portable head CT**
- Monitor for skin breakdown under energy transfer pads
- Maintain target temperature for at least 24 h

REWARMING

- Controlled rewarming at rate <0.4 °C/hr Rewarming >0.5°C/h can cause hypotension, electrolyte shifts, seizures, cerebral edema, and malignant arrhythmias
- Closely monitor electrolytes, particularly potassium and glucose
- Turn off sedation, analgesia, and neuromuscular blockade when patient's temperature reaches 98.6°F
- Maintain normothermia for at least 72 h
- Monitor neurologic exam and additional workup as indicated for prognostication

At any stage, STOP TTM if:

Patient consistently following commands
Severe life threatening hemorrhage
Severe hypotension or hemodynamically significant bradyarrhythmias*** despite maximal medical therapy

Figure 3.2 Implementation of therapeutic temperature management (TTM) after cardiac arrest

*Lactic acidosis is a normal physiologic response during hypothermia and may not be a reliable indicator of tissue perfusion

**Indications for urgent head CT include focal neurologic deficits, seizures, recent intracranial bleed, stroke, surgery or infection, or high risk for acute intracranial process (e.g. fall, anticoagulant use, recent brain surgery, known metastatic disease, known aneurysms, arteriovenous malformations, or other predisposing factors)
Indications for urgent continuous EEG monitoring is indicated if seizures at onset, prior history of seizures, clinical myoclonus or other jerking or seizure-like activity on examination

***For hemodynamically significant bradycardia, treatment options are isoproterenol or artificial pacing. Atropine is usually ineffective.

Two landmark clinical trials demonstrated that inducing mild-to-moderate hypothermia to 32 °–34 °C improved neurologically intact survival after out-of-hospital cardiac arrest due to witnessed ventricular fibrillation (VF).[6,7] The ideal duration and target temperature during TTM are the subject of debate. Nielsen et al. demonstrated no difference in neurologic outcome or mortality comparing TTM at 33 °C and 36 °C in a multicenter cohort of patients after out-of-hospital cardiac arrest (OHCA).[8] In a different study, patients treated at 36 °C demonstrated lower protocol adherence and a trend toward worse outcome, compared with historical controls treated at 33 °C, raising questions about the effectiveness and ease of implementation of TTM at 36 °C.[9] A retrospective cohort study of 782 comatose, adult OHCA patients found that patients treated during the targeted temperature management 33 °C period had higher odds of neurologically intact survival to hospital discharge compared with those treated during the targeted temperature management 36 °C period.[10]

One of the notable advantages of cooling to a relatively normal temperature includes lower sedative use for shivering and fewer systemic adverse effects related to hypothermia. A 36 °C goal particularly may be reasonable in patients with active noncompressible bleeding, hemodynamically significant bradyarrythmias, hypotension despite multiple pressor use, or presence of a significant infection, which may risk exacerbation at lower temperatures.

The optimal TTM duration remains debatable. While prolonged therapy up to 72 h is effective in newborns suffering from anoxic/hypoxic encephalopathy, TTM at 33 °C for 48 h did not significantly improve long-term neurological outcome when compared to 24 h duration in adult OHCA.[11]

At our institution, we recommend implementing TTM with a goal of 36 °C for 24 h from start of cooling process, followed by warming to 37 °C no faster than 0.5 °C per hour (Figure 3.3). After the first 24 h, we maintain normothermia at 37 °C until 72 h after arrest.

3.11.2   MONITORING THE PATIENT UNDERGOING TTM

If a decision to induce hypothermia is made, several physiologic factors must be taken into consideration.

-**Arrhythmias.** Cardiac conduction abnormalities, including bradycardia and QT prolongation, may occur during hypothermia. Sinus tachycardia or atrial fibrillation occurs frequently in mildly hypothermic patients. The risk of ventricular fibrillation increases at temperatures <30 °C. Arrhythmias in deeply hypothermic patients are difficult to treat, as the myocardium becomes less responsive to defibrillation and antiarrhythmic drugs. Interestingly, bradycardia during TTM at a temperature of 32–34 °C was more frequently associated with good neurologic outcome at discharge compared with nonbradycardic patients.[12] For hemodynamically significant bradycardia, isoproterenol is more likely to be helpful than atropine if needed. Mild hypothermia decreases cardiac output by about 25% and leads to increased vascular resistance and a rise in central venous pressure. During rewarming, cellular shifts can cause abrupt hyperkalemia with associated arrythmias.

-**Cold diuresis.** Acute cold stress reduces plasma volume and increases urine flow rate due to redistribution of plasma volume from the periphery to the central circulation in response to peripheral vasoconstriction. This "cold-diuresis" can cause hypovolemia and electrolyte abnormalities. Fluid repletion should be closely monitored. Hypo-osmolar fluids should be avoided to prevent exacerbation of cerebral edema. Electrolytes should be monitored every 4 h.

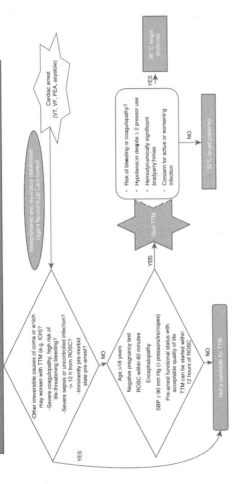

Figure 3.3 Post cardiac-arrest algorithm for patient selection for therapeutic temperature management (TTM)

-**Hypotension.** Retrospective reviews indicate that clinically significant hypotension was typically associated with temperatures of 32 °C, and with cooling for 48 h as compared with 24 h. While a decrease in mean arterial pressure (MAP) and cardiac output, and increase in vasopressor and inotrope use was observed, it was without deleterious effect on central venous oxygen saturation ($ScVO_2$). Lactic acidosis is commonly present and may not be a reliable indicator of tissue perfusion during hypothermia. Fluid repletion and maintenance of a MAP goal >65 mmHg or systolic BP goal >90 mmHg is essential. A higher goal of 80–100 mmHg may be indicated to optimize cerebral perfusion pressure, but this may be challenging to titrate as ICP monitoring is not routinely performed in post-cardiac arrest care.

-**Shivering.** Acute exposure to cold causes peripheral vasoconstriction, shivering, and increased metabolic heat production. Shivering, which primarily occurs during induction, can be highly detrimental as it increases oxygen consumption, prolongs the time to goal temperature, increases ICP and intraocular pressure, causes rhabdomyolysis, stretches surgical incisions and interrupts monitoring devices. It primarily occurs during induction. The Bedside Shivering Assessment Scale (BSAS) can be used to escalate treatments according to severity (Figure 3.4). Skin counterwarming can be performed by wrapping the head, neck, hands, and feet with blankets. Sedation with propofol, benzodiazepines, or fentanyl may be helpful. Magnesium helps lower shivering threshold. Opiates, in addition to their analgesic effects, can also help suppress shivering. Buspirone reduces the shivering threshold by 0.7 °C and may work synergistically with opioids. Neuromuscular blockade may be indicated if the above measures fail, but video EEG monitoring should be initiated as it suppresses convulsive movements. Meperidine can lower seizure threshold so is less favored.

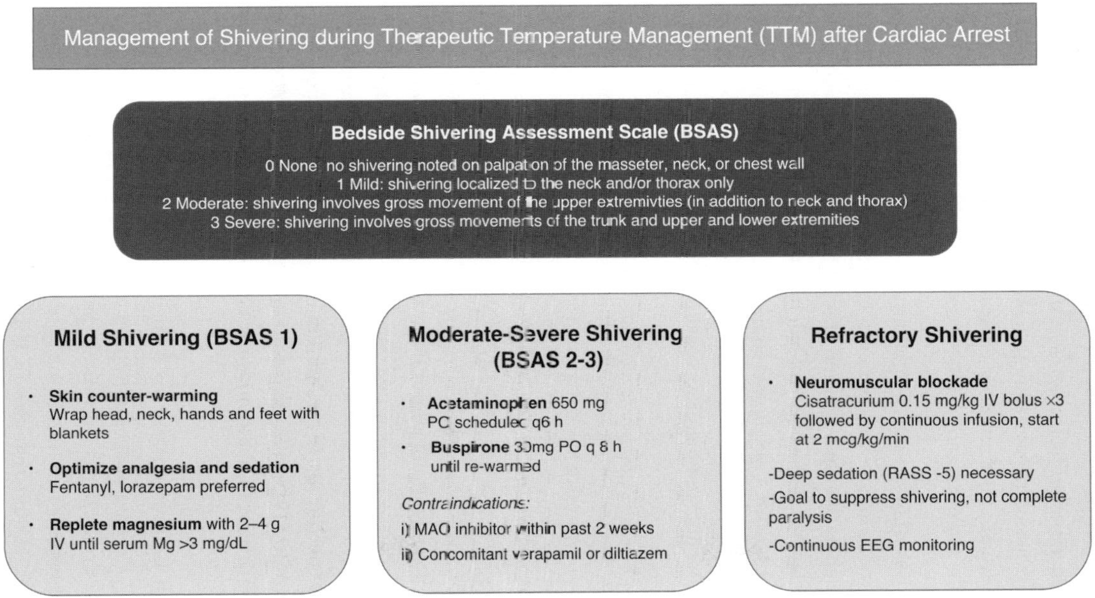

Management of Shivering during Therapeutic Temperature Management (TTM) after Cardiac Arrest

Bedside Shivering Assessment Scale (BSAS)

0 None: no shivering noted on palpation of the masseter, neck, or chest wall
1 Mild: shivering localized to the neck and/or thorax only
2 Moderate: shivering involves gross movement of the upper extremities (in addition to neck and thorax)
3 Severe: shivering involves gross movements of the trunk and upper and lower extremities

Mild Shivering (BSAS 1)

· **Skin counter-warming**
Wrap head, neck, hands and feet with blankets

· **Optimize analgesia and sedation**
Fentanyl, lorazepam preferred

· **Replete magnesium** with 2–4 g
IV until serum Mg >3 mg/dL

Moderate-Severe Shivering (BSAS 2-3)

· **Acetaminophen** 650 mg
PC schedule: q6 h

· **Buspirone** 30mg PO q 8 h
until re-warmed

Contraindications:
i) MAO inhibitor within past 2 weeks
ii) Concomitant verapamil or diltiazem

Refractory Shivering

· **Neuromuscular blockade**
Cisatracurium 0.15 mg/kg IV bolus ×3 followed by continuous infusion, start at 2 mcg/kg/min

-Deep sedation (RASS -5) necessary
-Goal to suppress shivering, not complete paralysis
-Continuous EEG monitoring

Figure 3.4 Management of shivering during therapeutic temperature management (TTM) after cardiac arrest

-**Mild coagulopathy.** TTM induces a mild coagulopathy due to its impact on coagulation factor activity and platelet function and the fibrinolytic system. Of note, platelet count and routine coagulation studies will usually be normal. If clinically significant bleeding occurs, rewarming to a temperature of 36 °C should be initiated.

-**Increased risk of infections.** Hypothermia impairs leukocyte function and, over periods longer than 24 h, can increase incidence of significant infections such as pneumonia when applied in ischemic stroke and TBI patients. A higher risk of wound infections, including pressure ulcers and catheter insertion sites, and impaired healing has also been reported. We recommend obtaining surveillance blood cultures in all patients 12 h after initiation of cooling and monitoring skin under cooling pads for breakdown.

-**Ventilation.** Arterial blood gas values need to be interpreted with care. PCO_2 may be 6–7 mmHg lower than that measured by blood gas sampling.

-**Drug metabolism** is decreased by hypothermia, and postanesthetic recovery may be prolonged. Fentanyl is a preferred analgesic, followed by lorazepam IV pushes. Midazolam has less reliable pharmacokinetics during hypothermia. Propofol use requires a 30% dose reduction due to accumulation during hypothermia. Signs and symptoms of propofol infusion syndrome (PRIS) should be carefully monitored for. The choice of sedatives and analgesia can be determined based on the need for antiepileptic effect (if post anoxic status epilepticus or myoclonic seizures present) and the use of neuromuscular blockade, which warrants deeper sedation.

-**Rewarming.** Common practice is to maintain a gradual rewarming rate of 0.25–0.5 °C/h. When hypothermia is prolonged, rewarming may be as gradual as 1 °C/day. Rapid rewarming can cause electrolyte abnormalities (e.g. hyperkalemia), cerebral edema, and seizures among other complications. In animal models of TBI, rewarming >0.5 °C/h eliminated the benefits of TTM. In experimental models of TBI and stroke, rapid rewarming was found to cause loss of cerebral autoregulation.

-**Post-rewarming.** Observational studies suggest that fever after rewarming is associated with worse neurologic outcomes. Active prevention of fever is reasonable in the post-rewarming phase.

-**Prognostication.** The bedside neurologic examination is unreliable for at least 72 h following resuscitation, even in the absence of TTM. Neurologic prognostication should not be performed prior to this timeframe. This may be delayed further accounting for sedation and other confounding factors.

3.11.3   ROLE OF THERAPEUTIC HYPOTHERMIA IN OTHER NEUROLOGIC CONDITIONS

TBI. Therapeutic hypothermia has demonstrated effectiveness in decreasing ICP but has not been convincingly shown to improve outcomes in TBI. Some systematic reviews and meta-analyses found an increased risk for pneumonia with induced hypothermia. In a 2015 trial, which evaluated hypothermia when added to other standard-of-care measures in patients with refractory intracranial hypertension within 10 days of TBI, no benefit was found but deaths and unfavorable outcomes were more common in the hypothermia group.[13]

Status Epilepticus. In a 2016 randomized trial of 270 patients, induced hypothermia showed no benefit when added to standard treatments for the initial treatment of convulsive status epilepticus. The rate of progression to EEG-confirmed status epilepticus on Day 1 was lower in the hypothermia group, but adverse events were also more frequent in this group.[14]

3.11.4   THERAPEUTIC INTERVENTIONS FOR TEMPERATURE MANAGEMENT

There is no consensus about the most effective method to deliver TTM and its impact on outcome. According to international guidelines, external or internal cooling devices can be used. Several devices are available for clinical use, with different technical characteristics, feasibility (i.e. in-hospital versus out-of-hospital), velocity to achieve target temperature, precision (i.e. maintenance of the target temperature within target ranges), invasiveness, potential side effects, and costs.[15]

3.11.4.1   Conventional Cooling Systems

Cold saline, crushed ice, or ice bags have the advantages of easy availability and low cost but are labor intensive and may not be as effective in maintaining target temperature.

3.11.4.2   Surface Cooling Systems

Surface cooling systems operate by circulating cold fluid or cold air through blankets or pads that are wrapped around the patient. A study comparing a water-circulating cooling blanket, to hydrogel-coated water-circulating energy transfer pads, showed that the pads were superior in controlling fever in critically ill neurologic patients. A study comparing the same surface system with an invasive intravascular system in post-cardiac arrest patients showed similar survival to hospital discharge and comparable neurologic function at follow-up.

The advantages with using surface systems are ease of application and rapid initiation of treatment. Most devices have computerized auto-feedback mechanisms allowing the user to set target temperature and the system modifies the water temperature using the feedback from patient's skin and core temperature sensors.

The disadvantages of these systems are rare risk of skin breakdown. The initiation of hypothermia varies between different devices and can range from 2 to 8 h. Maintenance of temperature may also be difficult. Shivering is more commonly seen with surface systems than with other systems, which may necessitate the use of additional medications.

3.11.4.3 Intravascular Cooling Systems

Intravascular cooling systems use percutaneously placed central venous catheters and circulate cool or warm saline in a closed loop through the catheter's balloon. The available systems have computerized temperature control with an auto-feedback mechanism and enable closely controlled temperature during maintenance and rewarming phases of temperature management. There are fewer incidences of failure to reach target temperature and less overcooling than with other systems and also less shivering compared to surface devices. There is an added risk of catheter-related bloodstream infection, venous thrombosis, and complications related to insertion of intravascular lines.

3.12 Upcoming Trials To Look Out for

- Influence of Cooling duration on Efficacy in Cardiac Arrest Patients (ICECAP) – randomized adaptive clinical trial to characterize the duration-response curve of induced hypothermia in comatose survivors of cardiac arrest and to determine the optimal duration of cooling.
- Targeted hypothermia versus targeted normothermia after out-of-hospital cardiac arrest (TTM2): A randomized clinical superiority trial. Target temperature of 33 °C after cardiac arrest will be compared with a strategy to maintain normothermia and early treatment of fever (≥37.8 °C).

References

1. O'Grady NP, Barie PS, Bartlett JG, et al. Guidelines for evaluation of new fever in critically ill adult patients: 2008 update from the American College of Critical Care Medicine and the Infectious Diseases Society of America. Crit Care Med. 2008;36:1330.

2. Benarroch E. Thermoregulation: recent concepts and remaining questions. Neurology. 2007;69:1293–97.

3. Dunkley EJC, Isbister GK, Sibbritt D, et al. The Hunter Serotonin Toxicity Criteria: simple and accurate diagnostic decision rules for serotonin toxicity. QJM-Int J Med. September 2003;96(9):635–42.

4. Baguley IJ, Perkes IE, Fernández-Ortega JF, et al. Paroxysmal sympathetic hyperactivity after acquired brain injury: consensus on conceptual definition, nomenclature, and diagnostic criteria. J Neurotrauma. 2014;31:1515–20.

5. Meyfroidt G, Baguley IJ, Menon DK. Paroxysmal sympathetic hyperactivity: the storm after acute brain injury. The Lancet Neurol. 2017;16(9):721–29.

6. The Hypothermia After Cardiac Arrest (HACA) Study Group. Mild therapeutic hypothermia to improve the neurologic outcome after cardiac arrest. N Engl J Med. 2002;346:549–56.

7. Bernard SA, Gray TW, Buist MD, et al. Treatment of comatose survivors of out-of-hospital cardiac arrest with induced hypothermia. N Engl J Med. 2002;346:557–63.

8. Nielsen N, Wetterslev J, Cronberg T, et al. Targeted temperature management at 33°C versus 36°C after cardiac arrest. N Engl J Med. December 5, 2013;369(23):2197–206.

9. Bray JE, Stub D, Bloom JE, et al. Changing target temperature from 33°C to 36°C in the ICU management of out-of-hospital cardiac arrest: a before and after study. Resuscitation. 2017;113:39–43.

10. Johnson NJ, Danielson KR, Counts CR, et al. Targeted temperature management at 33 versus 36 degrees: a retrospective cohort study. Crit Care Med. 2020;48:362–369.

11. Kirkegaard H, Søreide E, de Haas I, et al. Targeted temperature management for 48 vs 24 hours and neurologic outcome after out-of-hospital cardiac arrest: a randomized clinical trial. JAMA. 2017;318:341–50.

12. Stær-Jensen H, Sunde K, Olasveengen TM, et al. Bradycardia during therapeutic hypothermia is associated with good neurologic outcome in comatose survivors of out-of-hospital cardiac arrest. Crit Care Med. November 2014;42(11):2401–08.

13. Andrews PJ, Sinclair HL, Rodriguez A, et al. Hypothermia for intracranial hypertension after traumatic brain injury. N Engl J Med. 2015;373:2403.

14. Legriel S, Lemiale V, Schenck M, et al. Hypothermia for neuroprotection in convulsive status epilepticus. N Engl J Med. 2016;375:2457.

15. Vaity C, Al-Subaie N, Cecconi M. Cooling techniques for targeted temperature management post-cardiac arrest. Crit Care. 2015;19:103.

4

Approach to Neuroimaging of the Brain, Vessels, and Cerebral Edema

Muhammad Umair, Tyler Hinkel, Alexander W Korutz, Eric J Russell, and Alexander J Nemeth

Abstract

This introductory chapter on neuroradiology for neuro-critical care focuses on assessing appropriateness for reperfusion in the setting of acute ischemic stroke and discusses the imaging of acute intracranial hemorrhage and spinal cord injury.

4.1 Assessing Appropriateness for Reperfusion

Multiple trials published in 2015 demonstrated that improved outcomes could be obtained in appropriately selected ischemic stroke patients who underwent endovascular intervention with an attempt at reperfusion compared to those who did not. These trials included MR CLEAN, ESCAPE, EXTEND IA, SWIFT PRIME, and REVASCAT.[1,2] There are a variety of approaches to determine in any individual case the best therapeutic strategy, and neuroimaging plays an important role in these decisions.

4.1.1   THROMBOLYSIS

4.1.1.1   Intravenous Thrombolysis

Early trials of reperfusion therapy with intravenous thrombolysis demonstrated improved outcomes with reperfusion performed <3 h (and later up to 4 1/2 h) of symptom onset; however, reperfusion increases the risk of developing an intracranial hemorrhage by 10-fold. A notable limitation of IV thrombolysis centers on the fact that recanalization can only be obtained in at most 30% of patients with large vessel (ICA or proximal MCA) occlusion, and is most effective with more distal thrombi and emboli.[3]

4.1.1.2   Intra-arterial Thrombolysis

Intra-arterial thrombolysis involves direct infusion of a thrombolytic agent via a microcatheter that is placed near or into the site of arterial occlusion. Different thrombolytic agents can be infused (e.g. tPA). This technique can be combined with intravenous thrombolysis or with intra-arterial mechanical clot extraction, discussed later in this section.

Precise comparisons between IV and IA approaches to acute stroke are difficult to make due to differences in methods, patient populations, inclusion criteria, and so on.

Compared with IV thrombolysis, the rates of recanalization and reperfusion are significantly higher with intra-arterial thrombolysis, especially with large vessel occlusions, with demonstrated improved outcomes at 3-month follow-up. The recanalization rate for IA therapy was up to 66% compared to up to 30% for IV therapy.[4] IA thrombolysis had slightly better outcomes for patients with a Rankin score of 0–2 and excellent outcomes for those with a Rankin score of 0–1 when compared to IV thrombolysis administered within 3 h. Better outcomes were also observed compared to IV thrombolysis performed between 3 and 4.5 h.

When compared to controls only receiving intravenous heparin, there is a statistically significant increase in early hemorrhagic events among patients who receive intra-arterial thrombolysis; however, there is no significant difference in overall hemorrhagic events at 10 days between the two groups.[5]

4.1.1.3   Mechanical Thrombolysis

Intra-arterial mechanical thrombolysis can be performed when pharmacological thrombolysis is contraindicated, when pharmacologic thrombolysis fails to reestablish vessel patency, or if the presence of a large vessel occlusion reduces the efficacy of pharmacologic therapy alone. Mechanical thrombolysis performed alongside pharmacological thrombolysis may yield improved recanalization rates. Multiple techniques exist for mechanical thrombolysis, including clot extraction using snares/clot retrieval systems, balloon angioplasty, stenting, and clot maceration using catheters. Currently, there is evidence that mechanical thrombectomy may be more effective than IA tPA administration; however, future directions will likely be further defined by additional trials examining relative safety, feasibility, availability, expertise, and so forth.

4.1.2   CRITERIA FOR IA REPERFUSION

The following are the considerations for the use of IA reperfusion techniques; however, this may vary by case and institution.

1. Time window: With recent advancements, there is no strict time window. The true window depends on the adequacy of collateral circulation, and this can be assessed by functional neuroimaging protocols. Previously, a time window of <6 h from symptom onset was commonly used and may still be employed at some centers.

2. IA thrombolysis can be considered in cases where there is a contraindication to IV thrombolysis but not to IA thrombolysis (e.g. recent major surgery), or if the patient is outside a particular time window for IV thrombolysis (4 1/2 h from symptom onset). That said, an increasing number of institutions perform combined IV and

subsequent IA thrombolysis. Additionally, cases in which IV thrombolysis results in no significant improvement can be supplemented by IA thrombolysis.

3. Considerations for assessing the indications for IA thrombolysis/ thrombectomy:

   - A noninvasive vascular study, CTA or MRA, is highly recommended to identify the site of occlusion, and is often supplemented by perfusion CT or MR to evaluate hemodynamics and the adequacy of collateral circulation to define the presence of a viable therapeutic target (ischemic penumbra – defined as the difference between tissue at risk and tissue likely to be not salvageable).

   - Conventional catheter angiography may be performed to further define the vascular pathology to identify a therapeutic target, or as a prelude to intervention at the same sitting.

   - Therapeutic targets for IA therapy include the internal carotid arteries, the M1, and proximal M2 segments of the middle cerebral arteries, the vertebral arteries, and the basilar artery.

   - Detection of significant intracranial hemorrhage, mass effect, or the presence of an underlying tumor/mass by initial imaging may be a contraindication.

   - Identification of a large parenchymal core infarct on imaging with little, if any, ischemic penumbra would contraindicate intervention e.g. non-contrast CT demonstrating hypo-density or loss of gray–white differentiation for greater than one-third of MCA territory, non-contrast CT demonstrating an ASPECTS score <8, or MRI or CT perfusion imaging demonstrating little or no mismatch between ischemic brain at risk and core infarct.

   - No vascular imaging finding precluding access to the level of occlusion.

4. Availability of expertise at all levels and appropriate equipment on site.

Of note, the CLOTBUST (Combined Lysis Of Thrombus in Brain ischemia using Transcranial Ultrasound and Systemic T-PA) trial has shown superior rates of recanalization or clinical response with the use of combined IA and mechanical thrombolysis when compared to IA thrombolysis alone.

4.1.3 PERFUSION IMAGING

Patients with an acute infarct secondary to cerebral arterial occlusion must meet criteria to qualify for reperfusion therapy. Non-salvageable brain tissue is called "core infarct," while surrounding, still-viable tissue with decreased perfusion is called the "ischemic penumbra." The "ischemic penumbra" is the tissue that is potentially at risk and salvageable if an intervention is performed. The size of the core infarct relative to the ischemic penumbra helps determine which patients will benefit from intra-arterial interventions.

Although perfusion imaging can be performed with either CT or MRI, CT perfusion is often preferred in hyperacute situations, as this technique can be performed more rapidly with fewer logistical difficulties than MRI.

For perfusion imaging, the brain is imaged serially every 1–3 seconds during a contrast injection (iodinated contrast for CT or gadolinium based contrast for MR) at a rate of 4-5 ml/s to document contrast wash-in and wash-out. Total volume of blood per specific mass of brain (ml blood/100 g of brain tissue) is called cerebral blood volume (CBV) and is calculated as an area under the curve when attenuation in a particular voxel is plotted against time. Cerebral brain flow (CBF) is the amount of blood perfused per unit of time. The CBF is calculated by the slope of the upstroke of plot of change in contrast concentration against time. Mean transit time (MTT) is measured as the average transit time from arterial to venous system and generally ranges between 5 and 6 seconds. Traditionally, an MTT of >1.5 compared with a contralateral side voxel is considered prolonged and may suggest ischemia/penumbra. The relationship among CBV, CBF, and MTT can be described by the central volume principle.

$$CBF \ = CBV/MTT$$

$$CBV \ = CBF * MTT$$

$$MTT = CBV/CBF$$

Given a maintained blood volume, decreased cerebral flow results in increase in MTT and vice versa.

Time to peak (TTP) is another time factor that measures the time taken for contrast to achieve maximal enhancement in a voxel after injection. This includes any delays in arrival of contrast to the cerebral vasculature from extracranial factors. This delay can be accounted for by using an enhancement curve for a larger intracranial artery (called arterial input function) and the corrected output is called an impulse response function (IRF). Time to peak when adjusted for impulse response factor is called time to maximum (T-Max). Theoretically, T-Max should be close to 0 seconds in the setting of a normal blood supply and should be significantly increased in the setting of ischemia/infarction.

Increases in MTT or T-Max (delayed blood transit) are nonspecific and, therefore, cannot differentiate between regions of ischemia and core infarct. To differentiate between the two, CBV and CBF are evaluated in the region of delayed MTT or T-Max. Generally, an area contained within the region of delayed MTT with decreased CBV (representing collapse of the capillary bed in the ischemic zone) is considered ischemic core and the surrounding region with delayed MTT with normal or elevated CBV is considered ischemic penumbra, the latter potentially salvageable in the appropriately screened patient (Figure 4.1).

Although no strict cutoffs exist, generally favorable parameters for reperfusion are considered to be small core infarct when compared to the area of ischemic penumbra. A volumetric ratio of ischemic penumbra to core infarct (mismatch ratio) has been used as inclusion criteria for trials in the past (e.g. a mismatch ratio of 1.2 was used as inclusion criteria for the EXTEND IA trial and a mismatch ratio of 1.8 was used for the SWIFT PRIME trial). Additionally, patients with a core infarct of less than 70 ml

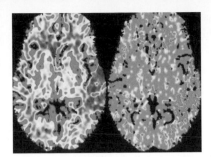

Figure 4.1 Perfusion imaging: Focal decrease in CBV (left) representing core infarct with a relatively larger area of increased MTT (right) that represents surrounding ischemic penumbra

were included in the EXTEND IA trial, while core infarct less than 50 ml was the inclusion criteria for the SWIFT PRIME trial. Currently, the use of these cutoffs is based on institutional experience and preference. Many institutions use semi-quantitative criteria of less than one-third of MCA territory core infarct or less than 70 ml of infarcted tissue seen on perfusion imaging as inclusion for a reperfusion attempt. In cases of nonavailability of perfusion imaging, MR diffusion imaging may be used as a substitute to evaluate the volume of core infarct and make decisions.

4.1.4   TICI SCALE TO ASSESS RESPONSE TO REPERFUSION

The clinical endpoint for success of a reperfusion attempt is evaluated with two main outcomes:

1. Recanalization: removal of physical blockage resulting in restoration of flow.
2. Reperfusion: restoration of flow downstream at the level of tissue/ capillaries. Reperfusion is a more important outcome as it defines the success of restoration of perfusion at the tissue level.

   To semi-quantitatively stratify the success of reperfusion intervention, the TICI scoring system was developed for cerebral reperfusion based on a similar system for coronary reperfusion called TIMI. The TICI score stratifies success in terms of recanalization and reperfusion of downstream tissue with better outcomes for a higher TICI score demonstrating a higher grade of reperfusion. For the majority of reperfusion interventions, procedural success to restore perfusion is commonly defined as an outcome TICI score of 2b or 3.

TICI Score:

0 = No perfusion

1 = Minimal or slow perfusion with penetration of occlusion

2 = Partial perfusion which may be contrast opacification past obstruction with either a slower rate of flow distal to the obstruction compared to contralateral side and/or slower rate of contrast clearance from distal bed compared to contralateral side

2a = Less than two-thirds of total vascular territory is opacified

2b = Complete filling of vascular territory, at a slower rate than normal

3 = Complete perfusion

4.2 Acute Intracranial Hemorrhage

Acute intracranial hemorrhage is treated as an emergency as timely intervention may prevent significant morbidity or mortality.[6] Given the rigid, noncompliant nature of the calvarium, a small volume of hemorrhage can trigger significant elevations of intracranial pressure and may result in a herniation syndrome. Direct injury of the brain parenchyma may be compounded by vascular compression related to brain swelling, leading to secondary acute infarction. Alteration of CSF flow dynamics can also lead to acute obstructive hydrocephalus. In addition to these direct pressure-related complications, additional consequences/complications can lead to hemodynamic collapse or compromise due to autonomic dysfunction (e.g. Cushing reflex).

4.2.1   TRAUMATIC ACUTE INTRACRANIAL HEMORRHAGE

Acute intracranial hemorrhage can be classified by both mechanism (traumatic or nontraumatic/spontaneous) and location (intraparenchymal, subarachnoid/intraventricular, subdural, and epidural).

4.2.1.1   Extra-Axial Hemorrhage

Subdural Hemorrhage

Subdural hemorrhage (SDH) refers to a collection of blood within the potential subdural space. The majority of these hematomas arise from a venous source secondary to torsional shear injury of the bridging veins or from cortical vein injury from a depressed fracture. Rarely, SDH can result from an arterial bleed from a calvarial fracture. SDH is typically crescentic in shape; however, rarely, if small, or in the setting of volume loss or rapid accumulation, they can assume a lentiform shape. By definition, SDH is contained by dural reflections such as the interhemispheric falx and tentorial leaflets. As a result, these collections usually do not cross midline, in contradistinction to collections in the epidural space.

Although SHD is typically hyperdense relative to adjacent CSF and brain parenchyma on CT, if hyperacute, in the setting of coagulopathy/anemia or if rapidly expanding, hyperdense SDH may be hard to separate from the overlying calvarium with standard "brain" window viewing settings. It is for this reason that "wider" window settings (e.g. liver windows) are also utilized as part of the routine search pattern to evaluate for SDH.

SDH may have interspersed hypodense/isodense components. This latter scenario can create a diagnostic dilemma, as mixed density hematoma may also be the result of acute hemorrhage into a subacute/chronic collection. Also, subacute SDH may be in whole or in part isodense relative to parenchyma and as a result may be difficult to visualize.

SDH decreases in attenuation with time, eventually becoming hypodense to brain tissue when chronic. Posttraumatic subdural fluid collections secondary to an arachnoid tear that allows for CSF leakage into the subdural space are hypodense to brain (CSF density) and are termed subdural hygroma. These collections are common among older patients, often appearing days after injury. These are usually asymptomatic and resolve spontaneously.

Larger SDHs with accompanying mass effect/herniation result in ICU admission for ICP monitoring and possible neurosurgical intervention. Smaller hematomas without significant mass effect can be followed conservatively. Subdural hematomas that persist or recur after treatment can be treated with middle meningeal artery embolization as devascularization may prevent further leakage into the collection.

Epidural Hemorrhage

Epidural hematoma (EDH) is an uncommon entity whereby blood collects between the skull and the layers of the dura. These usually result from an arterial bleed (e.g. middle meningeal arterial laceration in the setting of a squamosal temporal bone fracture). EDHs expand rapidly under higher pressure and may rapidly produce brain herniation. Less commonly, laceration of a dural venous sinus can cause a lower pressure venous epidural that expands relatively slowly. In such cases, careful analysis of the imaging studies may identify the site of venous disruption.

On CT, acute EDH is hyperdense relative to brain and assumes a lentiform shape. Density variations may occur in cases of hyperacute hemorrhage, active hemorrhage, and coagulopathies. Active bleeding into a hyperacute EDH may result in lower density areas within the collection, since new unclotted blood is less dense than more concentrated blood clot (the swirl sign). While SDHs are usually bound by dural reflections and do cross the falx or tentorium, EDHs may do so by displacing the dura inward. EDH will not track along the tentorium. However, exceptions to these rules exist. For instance, in some circumstances, the high-pressure hemorrhage and complex fractures associated with epidural hematomas result in extension across suture lines, especially in pediatric patients.

Due to the propensity for rapid expansion, EDH is often followed closely with CT imaging in an ICU setting. Surgical intervention, if necessary, is based on the patient's symptoms and imaging findings.

Subarachnoid Hemorrhage

Subarachnoid hemorrhage (SAH) is blood within the CSF-containing subarachnoid spaces (spaces between the brain surface/pia mater and arachnoid mater) and extends into the cerebral sulci, fissures, and basilar cisterns. The majority of SAHs are secondary to trauma or a ruptured aneurysm; however, less common causes of SAH include benign perimesencephalic hemorrhage of presumed venous origin (Figure 4.2), ruptured arteriovenous malformation/dural arteriovenous fistula, ruptured mycotic aneurysm, reversible cerebral vasoconstrictive

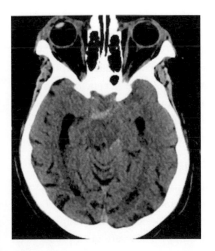

Figure 4.2 Perimesencephalic subarachnoid hemorrhage (SAH) of presumed venous etiology demonstrating layering blood in the suprasellar cistern

syndrome, cerebral amyloid angiopathy, vasculitis, and intracranial arterial dissection.[7] In traumatic SAH, the etiology is rupture of vessels in the subarachnoid space or spillage of hemorrhage from parenchymal contusion.

On CT, acute SAH is hyperdense to brain and CSF. On MRI, acute SAH is typically hyperintense on FLAIR, mildly hyperintense to CSF on T1, and demonstrates low signal and blooming artifact on T2 gradient echo (GRE) or susceptibility-weighted imaging (SWI), although T2* hypointensity may be less with SAH than that seen in parenchymal bleeds due to the high oxygen content of CSF resulting in less complete formation of the deoxyhemoglobin that serves as its basis. With subsequent oxidation of hemoglobin to methemoglobin, SAH becomes hyperintense to brain on T1-weighted images.

In cases in which SAH is still suspected despite a negative head CT (and MRI, if performed), lumbar puncture may be helpful, although the time window is generally limited due to clearance of breakdown products of hemoglobin from the CSF spaces. In the chronic phase, MRI often demonstrates T2* hypointensity due to the formation of superficial hemosiderin staining of the brain surface and leptomeninges (superficial siderosis) in areas of prior SAH. In both the acute and chronic phases, SAH can be associated with the development of hydrocephalus due to subarachnoid adhesions, resulting in obstruction of CSF resorption. In days following initial bleeding, patients should be screened for the development of arterial vasospasm resulting from the presence of blood adjacent to the arteries, a secondary complication that can lead to ischemia with significant morbidity and mortality.

4.2.1.2   Intra-axial Hemorrhage

Accumulation of blood within brain parenchyma can be secondary to traumatic or nontraumatic causes. Hemorrhagic parenchymal contusions typically occur at the direct site of impact (coup) or directly opposite to impact (contrecoup). These are most pronounced in the anterior/inferior frontal lobes and the anterior/inferior temporal lobes, and also the occipital poles, secondary to skull geometry in these regions.

On CT, parenchymal contusions often contain areas of hyperdense petechial hemorrhage along the axis of mechanical injury with surrounding parenchymal edema. On MRI, as discussed earlier, hemorrhage has a variable appearance depending on the time passed after extravasation. Hyperacute hemorrhage is hardest to identify, as T1 images show slight hyperintensity to brain as a proteinaceous fluid without marked T1 hyperintensity that develops later as blood oxidizes to methemoglobin, and T2 hyperintensity before deoxyhemoglobin forms to cause T2/T2* shortening (low signal on these sequences). With time, hemorrhage resorbs leaving regional encephalomalacia/gliosis often with residual hemosiderin staining (only visible on MRI).

Post-traumatic parenchymal hemorrhage may also occur in the setting of diffuse axonal injury (DAI), whereby the brain experiences multifocal shear injury from rotational acceleration/deceleration forces that occur at sites where adjacent regions of have different specific gravities with disruption of the gray–white junction. Resultant injuries are therefore most pronounced at the gray–white interfaces, between white matter bundles within the corpus callosum and in more severe cases, within the brain stem.

In cases of acute DAI, CT may be unrevealing (unless there are other accompanying intracranial traumatic findings such as SDH or larger parenchymal hematomas) or present as subtle areas of petechial hemorrhage in typical locations. On MRI, hemorrhagic lesions associated with DAI will be seen as multifocal sites of low T2 and T2* signal (hypo-intensity) at the gray–white interfaces and/or within the corpus callosum/brain stem on T2 GRE or SWI. These sequences, however, are insensitive to nonhemorrhagic shear injuries, which may be more numerous and are best detected acutely on diffusion-weighted MR imaging (DWI).

Acute parenchymal contusions and hematomas are associated with complications related to regional mass effect.[8] It is for these reasons that patients are closely monitored in an ICU setting along with serial imaging to detect delayed expansion of hemorrhages, worsening edema, secondary infarction, and when necessary, intracranial pressure monitoring.[9] Neurosurgical intervention may be pursued in the setting of rapidly increasing intracranial pressure.

4.2.2 NONTRAUMATIC/SPONTANEOUS INTRACRANIAL HEMORRHAGE

Nontraumatic/spontaneous hemorrhage is common in both the subarachnoid and intraparenchymal spaces, with common etiologies including ruptured aneurysm, hypertensive hemorrhage, hemorrhagic transformation of an acute infarct, hemorrhagic neoplasm, benign perimesencephalic hemorrhage, hemorrhage secondary to arteriovenous malformation/dural arteriovenous-fistula/cavernous-malformation, cerebral amyloid angiopathy, vasculitis, and reversible cerebral vasoconstriction syndrome.

Non-contrast CT is the first modality used to detect the bleed, with further characterization by MRI, CTA, MRA, or conventional angiography to evaluate extent and etiology.

Specific management goals for spontaneous intracranial hemorrhage depend on the underlying etiology. Similar to other types of intracranial hemorrhage, acute management (i.e. surgical versus conservative) is determined by the size of the hemorrhage (degree of mass effect and accompanying mass effect-related complications such as herniation, elevated ICP, and hydrocephalus) as well as the change in hematoma size over time. In the literature, outcomes depend upon the volume of hematoma, which can be calculated using the formula for the volume of an ellipsoid ($0.52 \times AP \times CC \times TV$), also known as the ABC/2 method.

4.2.2.1 Intracranial Aneurysm Rupture

The most common cause of nontraumatic SAH is intracranial aneurysm. Aneurysms are eccentric dilatations from the side walls of arteries, predominantly occurring at vascular branching points. These most commonly occur at the circle of Willis, including the internal carotid artery origin of the posterior communicating artery, along the anterior communicating artery complex involving the junction with anterior cerebral artery (ACA) A1 and A2 segments, and at the bifurcation of the MCA M1 segment. Posterior fossa aneurysms are common at the basilar artery terminus or at the origin of the posterior inferior cerebellar artery. Aneurysms that are increasing in size, developing adjacent "daughter sacs" (Murphy's tit) or that are associated with enhancement of the aneurysm wall (inflammation) are associated with a higher risk of rupture. In the case of multiple aneurysms, the one that has bled is often the largest aneurysm present, and may be associated with wall irregularity and adjacent subarachnoid clot.

Non-contrast CT is the initial test of choice. In hemorrhage that is localized, the epicenter of the hemorrhage may suggest the location of rupture (e.g. sylvian fissure in MCA-bifurcation aneurysm or lateral suprasellar cistern for posterior communicating artery aneurysm). The aneurysm may be detected on CT as a lower density filling defect in the subarachnoid blood if large enough. Ultimately, CTA, MRA, or conventional angiography is performed to define the aneurysm and parent artery anatomy and for interventional planning (open surgical clipping or endovascular coiling and flow diversion).

Similar to other types of intracranial hemorrhage, patients with aneurysmal SAH are monitored closely in an ICU setting with serial imaging.

4.2.2.2 Hypertensive Intracranial Hemorrhage

Uncontrolled hypertension results in small vessel lipo-hyalinosis/microaneurysm formation as well as accelerated large vessel atherosclerosis. Rupture of these microaneurysms/weakened vessel

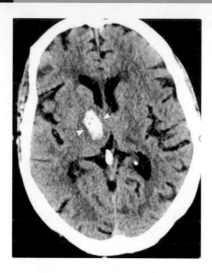

Figure 4.3 Right thalamocapsular hemorrhage secondary to hypertensive emergency, seen as hyperdensity on non-contrast head CT

walls results in hypertensive hemorrhage. While diagnosis can be straightforward in the setting of hypertensive crisis/emergency with a typical central intraparenchymal hemorrhage, diagnosis of a hypertensive etiology may be a diagnosis of exclusion after other etiologies have been ruled out. The distribution in the basal ganglia, cerebellum, and pons helps differentiate from the lobar pattern of hemorrhage seen in cerebral amyloid angiopathy (Figure 4.3). Intraventricular extension is more common as well due to central location with risk for hydrocephalus development.

Management is ICU level of care with serial CT imaging, with possible CTA, MRA, or catheter angiography to rule out active hemorrhage (seen on CTA or MRA as punctate focus of active hemorrhage called the spot sign) or an underlying vascular lesion.[10] Contrast-enhanced MRI can provide additional information regarding chronic micro-bleeds in chronic uncontrolled hypertension (central distribution) or cerebral amyloid angiopathy (lobar distribution).

4.2.2.3   Cerebral Amyloid Angiopathy

Cerebral amyloid angiopathy (CAA) is typically a disease of normotensive elderly patients whereby amyloid proteins are deposited in the walls of the vasculature. Clinically, patients with CAA can present either with peripheral lobar hemorrhage or with convexity SAH. Very commonly, patients with CAA will have accompanying findings of numerous chronic micro-bleeds that demonstrate a peripheral distribution. Similar to chronic microhemorrhage in other diseases, these findings are best visualized on T2* (GRE) or susceptibility-weighted imaging (SWI).

4.2.2.4   Hemorrhagic Transformation of an Acute Infarct

Acute ischemic infarcts are at risk for intra-parenchymal hemorrhage secondary to vessel wall fragility (hemorrhagic transformation). Hemorrhagic transformation often occurs beginning around day 2 but can occur earlier with larger infarcts, prior thrombolysis (IA > IV), or in the setting of an underlying coagulopathy.

As described earlier, the appearance of hemorrhage varies very dramatically depending on the age of the blood.

4.2.2.5   Cerebral Venous Infarct

Thrombosis of the dural venous sinuses or superficial/deep cerebral veins can occur in the setting of hypercoagulable disorders, dehydration, oral contraceptive use, pregnancy, thrombophilia, collagen vascular disease, hyperviscosity syndromes (e.g. sickle cell disease, myeloma), trauma, or neoplasm. Venous occlusion leads to upstream vascular congestion, edema, blood-brain barrier breakdown, and petechial and/or gross hemorrhage.

Patients suspected of having venous thrombosis are often first evaluated with a non-contrast CT, and the parenchyma may be initially normal. In some patients, parenchymal edema/hemorrhage due to venous congestion may appear in a pattern that is not typical for arterial occlusion. A key finding on non-contrast CT is hyperdensity along the course of the involved vein/sinus. The location of edema/hemorrhage on CT may direct an observer to the location of the thrombosed vessel (e.g. temporal lobe hemorrhage in the setting of Vein of Labbe occlusion, thalamic edema with internal cerebral vein thrombosis, and bi-hemispheric hemorrhage at the vertex in a patient with superior sagittal sinus occlusion). On conventional MRI, the involved vein/sinus may demonstrate loss of the normal flow void best seen on T2 imaging. Ultimately, CT and MR venography are the diagnostic tests of choice for evaluation of venous occlusion. These studies will demonstrate a total or incomplete lack of flow signal or enhancement within the involved vessel.

The management of dural venous thrombosis involves systemic anticoagulation, hydration, and alleviation of modifiable risk factors (e.g. stopping OCP, managing thrombophilia), and in limited circumstances, interventional recanalization of a thrombosed venous sinus.

4.2.3   BRIEF REVIEW OF IMAGING MODALITIES TO ASSESS ACUTE INTRA-CRANIAL HEMORRHAGE

4.2.3.1   Non-contrast Head CT

Non-contrast CT is usually the first test ordered to establish the diagnosis of acute hemorrhage and hemorrhage-related complications (e.g. herniation, hydrocephalus, secondary infarction). Once the initial diagnosis is established, serial imaging with non-contrast CT can be used for follow-up as well.

4.2.3.2   CTA/MRA

In the acute setting, most patients with nontraumatic hemorrhage are evaluated with CTA of the head and neck to evaluate for a potential source of hemorrhage (e.g. aneurysm, vascular malformation, vasculitis) as well as the possibility of active bleeding (aka "spot sign"). MRA of the head and neck with and without contrast is an alternative. MRA can also be performed without contrast if contrast is contraindicated (e.g. pregnant patient): however, non-contrast MRA in the cervical region is more often degraded by motion artifact compared with dynamic contrast enhanced MRA. Non-contrast black-blood MRA of the neck vasculature is also under investigation and may eventually obviate the need for contrast-enhanced studies.

4.2.3.3   CT and MR Venography

CTV and MRV are effective for the diagnosis of dural sinus and cerebral venous thrombosis. Both techniques are best performed with contrast during a phase of imaging that optimally opacifies the venous structures; however, non-contrast MRV can be used when contrast is contraindicated, although it is more prone to artifact. On contrast-enhanced CTV and MRV, a venous thrombus typically presents as a central filling defect within the venous structure, with enhancement of the dural margin and possible expansion of the vessel lumen (Figure 4.4).

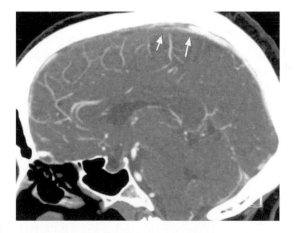

Figure 4.4 Thrombus occluding the superior sagittal sinus anteriorly with patent sinus posteriorly seen on this mid-sagittal image demonstrating venous sinus thrombosis

4.2.3.4   MRI

Conventional structural brain imaging with MRI is indicated in multiple situations. Most commonly, a "tumor protocol" with contrast-enhanced MRI and 3D volumetric post-contrast imaging is performed in a patient with nontraumatic parenchymal hemorrhage and no clear underlying cause on CTA in order to exclude an underlying mass or infarct. MRI can also be performed in cases when there is clinical concern for subtle hemorrhage such as SAH that is not identified on CT, as FLAIR sequences are quite sensitive. Finally, MRI can be performed if there is an equivocal focus of hemorrhage versus artifact that is questioned on a non-contrast CT and the MRI is then utilized to assess whether this was a true finding. In the setting of hemorrhage versus artifact on an initial CT, a short-term follow-up CT (e.g. 6 h) can also be performed to see if the finding persists or goes away, the latter suggesting either artifact or hemorrhage that has resolved.

4.3 Spinal Cord Injury

Spinal trauma that results in instability that can rapidly lead to extrinsic compression of the spinal cord can result in poor patient outcomes that can be avoided with accurate and fast diagnosis. Knowledge of the strengths and limitations of imaging modalities allows for more accurate diagnosis and timely coordination with care teams. Computed tomography (CT) and magnetic resonance imaging (MRI) are crucial tools in order to confirm injury location, delineate the extent of injury, and assess for the possibility of spine instability and/or neural compromise[11] (Figure 4.5). This brief guide will cover the strengths and limitations of both imaging modalities as well as when it is appropriate to perform these examinations.

The National Emergency X-Radiography Utilization Study (NEXUS) is a clinical tool that helps determine the appropriateness of imaging after

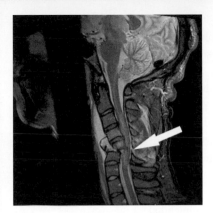

Figure 4.5 The T2-weighted sagittal scan demonstrates a three column, unstable flexion teardrop fracture involving the C5 vertebral body with retropulsion of bone into the spinal canal. There is severe spinal canal stenosis and cord compression, and extensive central cord T2 hyperintensity representing diffuse cord edema from C3 to C6. Focal low signal in this edema field likely represents hemorrhage, a poor prognostic finding (white arrow)

initial presentation. This tool uses five clinical factors that are each associated with an increased risk for spinal cord injury, with studies showing high sensitivity rates for NEXUS as a clinical tool. Canadian Cervical Rules (CCR) have also been used to evaluate cervical spine injury with similar sensitivities.[12]

The Congress of Neurological Surgeons and the American College of Radiology have developed thorough guidelines for the appropriateness of utilizing certain imaging modalities to assess acute cervical spine and spinal cord injuries. After determining that spinal imaging is necessary for a patient utilizing either NEXUS or CCR, providers should use the American College of Radiology appropriateness criteria in order to determine the best imaging modality to address the clinical question.

4.3.1 COMPUTED TOMOGRAPHY

CT is widely available and typically the first study employed to rapidly assess acute osseous injury and possible spinal canal compromise, and is the gold standard to determine instability. In the setting of trauma, CT has been shown to be superior to radiographs for the detection of acute fractures.[13]

Important limitations of CT include the inability of CT to directly screen for ligamentous injury as well as injury to the substance of the spinal cord that cannot be immediately inferred from critical narrowing of the osseous spinal canal. For this reason, MRI is often obtained after CT to evaluate the spinal cord, ligaments, intervertebral disks and paraspinal soft tissues. In controlled circumstances with a clinician present, flexion and extension radiographs may be performed to assess stability without compromising neurological function in neurologically intact patients.

Both the ACR and Congress of Neurologic Surgeons agree that radiographic evaluation is not recommended for the awake, asymptomatic patient without neck pain or tenderness and a normal neurological examination.

4.3.1.1   Following the ACR Appropriateness Criteria (2018)

CT of the cervical spine without IV contrast: Indications include patients 16 years and older who meet NEXUS or CCR criteria with suspected acute blunt trauma or findings of spine injury on radiograph.

CT angiography neck: Indicated for patients with suspected spine blunt trauma with clinical or imaging findings concerning for arterial injury, prior positive imaging is not required prior to utilizing this imaging modality if there is high clinical concern.

4.3.2   MAGNETIC RESONANCE IMAGING

The main indications for MRI in spinal trauma include evaluation for cord injury, CT findings suggestive of ligamentous injury (prevertebral hematoma, spondylolisthesis, asymmetric disk space widening, facet widening/dislocations), evaluation for causes of cord impingement (hematoma, disk herniation), evaluation for vascular injury and delineating between acute and chronic fractures.

A typical MRI protocol to assess for spinal injuries include Axial T1, T2, T2*, and Sagittal T1, T2 T2*GRE, and STIR sequences. MRI should be performed within 72 h of the injury to ensure edema is conspicuous on fluid sensitive sequences. High-resolution proton density and GRE sequences may also be obtained through the C1–C2 level to evaluate the integrity of the ligaments at the craniocervical junction.[14] MRI is the imaging modality of choice for detection of soft tissue and spinal cord injuries as well as predicting prognosis of spinal cord injuries. The MR detection of areas of traumatic hemorrhage within an edematous area of cord contusion, in a patient with paraplegia or quadriplegia, suggests a poorer prognosis for functional recovery than nonhemorrhagic contusion. MRA may also be employed when vascular injury (e.g. arterial dissection) is suspected clinically.

Although MRI is very sensitive for detecting soft tissue abnormalities and edema, there are limitations of this modality. First, MRI examinations require a significant amount of time to complete compared to CT and may not be suitable for the unconscious or unstable patient. Second, metallic susceptibility artifact from surgical hardware, implantable devices and metallic foreign bodies can significantly limit these examinations and decrease the sensitivity of MRI to detect traumatic injury.

4.3.2.1 Following the ACR Appropriateness Criteria

MRI without contrast is indicated in patients 16 or older with suspected or confirmed cervical spinal cord or nerve root injury or high clinical concern suggestive of ligamentous injury after CT is obtained. In obtunded patients, MRI can be obtained after CT to evaluate for soft tissue injuries.[15]

MRA neck with and without IV contrast should be obtained in patients with blunt trauma with high clinical concern or imaging findings suggestive of arterial injury. Axial fat-saturated sequences should be included.

When evaluating a patient with a suspected traumatic injury of the spine, tools like NEXUS and CCR can help assess the need for imaging.

Once the need for imaging has been confirmed, the physical exam and clinical evaluation for suspected injury (i.e. likelihood of osseous injury, ligamentous injury, or spinal cord trauma) will dictate what the appropriate next step should be.

References

1. Goyal M, Demchuk AM, Menon BK, Eesa M, Rempel JL, Thornton J, Roy D, Jovin TG, Willinsky RA, Sapkota BL. Randomized assessment of rapid endovascular treatment of ischemic stroke. N Engl J Med. 2015;372(11):1019–30.

2. Campbell BC, Mitchell PJ, Kleinig TJ, Dewey HM, Churilov L, Yassi N, Yan B, Dowling RJ, Parsons MW, Oxley TJ. Endovascular therapy for ischemic stroke with perfusion-imaging selection. N Engl J Med. 2015;372(11):1009–18.

3. Hacke W, Kaste M, Fieschi C, von Kummer R, Davalos A, Meier D, Larrue V, Bluhmki E, Davis S, Donnan G. Randomised double-blind placebo-controlled trial of thrombolytic therapy with intravenous alteplase in acute ischaemic stroke (ECASS II). Lancet. 1998;352(9136):1245–51.

4. Furlan A, Higashida R, Wechsler L, Gent M, Rowley H, Kase C, Pessin M, Ahuja A, Callahan F, Clark WM. Intra-arterial prourokinase for acute ischemic stroke: the PROACT II study: a randomized controlled trial. JAMA. 1999;282(21):2003–11.

5. Lee M, Hong K-S, Saver JL. Efficacy of intra-arterial fibrinolysis for acute ischemic stroke: meta-analysis of randomized controlled trials. Stroke. 2010;41(5):932–37.

6. Hemphill III JC, Greenberg SM, Anderson CS, Becker K, Bendok BR, Cushman M, Fung GL, Goldstein JN, Macdonald RL, Mitchell PH. Guidelines for the management of spontaneous intracerebral hemorrhage: a guideline for healthcare professionals from the American Heart Association/American Stroke Association. Stroke. 2015;46(7):2032–60.

7. Macellari F, Paciaroni M, Agnelli G, Caso V. Neuroimaging in intracerebral hemorrhage. Stroke. 2014;45(3):903–08.

8. Mendelow AD, Gregson BA, Rowan EN, Murray GD, Gholkar A, Mitchell PM, Investigators SI. Early surgery versus initial conservative treatment in patients with spontaneous supratentorial lobar intracerebral haematomas (STICH II): a randomised trial. The Lancet. 2013;382(9890):397–408.

9. Garg RK, Liebling SM, Maas MB, Nemeth AJ, Russell EJ, Naidech AM. Blood pressure reduction, decreased diffusion on MRI, and outcomes after intracerebral hemorrhage. Stroke. 2012;43(1):67–71.

10. Wada R, Aviv RI, Fox AJ, Sahlas DJ, Gladstone DJ, Tomlinson G, Symons SP. CT angiography "spot sign" predicts hematoma expansion in acute intracerebral hemorrhage. Stroke. 2007;38(4):1257–62.

11. Kumar Y, et al. Role of magnetic resonance imaging in acute spinal trauma: a pictorial review. BMC Musculoskeletal Disorders. 2016;17:310.

12. Hoffman JR, et al. Validity of a set of clinical criteria to rule out injury to the cervical spine in patients with blunt trauma. National Emergency X-Radiography Utilization Study Group. N Engl J Med. July 13, 2000;343(2):94–99.

13. Shah L, et al. Imaging of spine trauma. Neurosurgery. 2016;79:626–42.

14. Miyanji F, et al. Acute cervical traumatic spinal cord injury: MR imaging findings correlated with neurologic outcome – prospective study with 100 consecutive patients. Radiology. 2007; 243(3):820–27.

15. American College of Radiology. ACR Appropriateness Criteria: suspected spine trauma. Available from: www.acr.org.

5

Airway and Ventilator Management of the Neurologically Critically Ill Patient

Howard Lee and Michael L Ault

Abstract

Airway and ventilator management of the neurologically critically ill population poses several specific challenges for providers. These include the prevention of further injury due to hemodynamic instability or hypoxia; understanding the indications for tracheal intubation such as the need for invasive mechanical ventilation, upper airway obstruction, bronchial hygiene, and inability to protect airway; and securing airway in a rapid fashion to prevent aspiration. These patients typically do not have issues with lung mechanics, rather they have issues with airway protection and management of bronchial secretions. Depending on the neurologic pathology, these patients may require tracheostomy.

5.1 Airway and Ventilator Management of the Neurologic Critically Ill Patient

This chapter briefly reviews airway and ventilator management in the neurologic critically ill patient. Neurologic injuries and pathologies can pose devastating sequelae for afflicted patients and necessitate an artificial airway for mechanical ventilation. The categorization of neurologic pathologies can be generalized into either central or peripheral pathologies.

Central pathologies including traumatic brain injury (TBI), stroke, intracranial bleeding, elevated ICP, and intoxications can lead to impairment of consciousness, respiratory drive, and protective airway reflexes. Impaired consciousness, typically due to disruption of either cerebral hemisphere or the reticular activation system, can lead to aspiration and death. In the trauma patient population, a severe level of impaired consciousness is defined as a Glasgow Coma Score (GCS) ≤ 8. The respiratory center, located within the pons and medulla, controls respiratory drive. Disruptions can lead to pathological breathing patterns as well as respiratory failure. Additionally, impaired consciousness or injury to the brain stem can cause bulbar dysfunction leading to the loss of protective airway reflexes such as cough, gag, and swallowing. Swallowing is a complex reflex that involves the coordination of several oropharyngeal structures such as closure of the glottis, elevation of the larynx, and a transient cessation of respiration. Neurologic injury that impairs swallowing can lead to macro/micro aspiration.

Peripheral pathologies lead to the impairment of respiratory mechanics. Peripheral lesions that lead to respiratory failure include pathologies of the anterior horn (ALS, polio, cervical spine injuries), motor nerve (GBS), and the neuromuscular junction (myasthenia gravis). Normal diaphragm function accounts for approximately 70–80% of ventilatory function. Other muscles such as intercostal and scalene muscles also assist in ventilation. Patients who present with peripheral pathologies that involve these muscle groups can develop respiratory failure due to ineffective alveolar gas exchange. Peripheral pathologies impacting muscles of respiration as well as abdominal muscles can lead to an ineffective cough. An ineffective cough prevents bronchial secretion clearance and may lead to aspiration, pneumonia, and eventually respiratory failure. Additionally, bulbar dysfunction can lead to discordant swallowing and aspiration.

Both central and peripheral neurologic pathologies may call for an artificial airway and mechanical ventilation.

5.1.1   AIRWAY MANAGEMENT

Understanding the general principles of airway management is essential in the care of patients who are critically ill. These same principles apply to the neurologic critically ill. Providers can use high-flow nasal cannula (HFNC) to support patients with hypoxemia. Noninvasive positive pressure ventilation (NIPPV), such as BiPAP or average volume-assured pressure support (AVAPS), can be used to support patients with hypoventilation. If noninvasive measures fail, patients will require placement of an artificial airway and mechanical ventilation.

The placement of an artificial airway should be done in a systematic fashion. If time permits, review of the patient's history, airway history, airway examination, imaging studies and assessment of the patient's level of cooperation/consciousness should occur. In emergency settings, orotracheal intubation is preferred as it is faster than nasotracheal intubation. Patients who present in cardiac arrest should undergo emergency tracheal intubation. In patients who have sustained traumatic injuries, a concomitant cervical spine injury should be suspected, and appropriate precautions to protect the cervical spine during tracheal intubation should be used.

5.1.1.1   Indications for Intubation

The decision to intubate should be made if any of the following occur: inadequate ventilation/oxygenation with noninvasive measures, upper airway obstruction, inadequate bronchial hygiene, and/or the patient's inability to protect their airway (Table 5.1). Patients with impending respiratory failure who can no longer be supported with noninvasive measures should be intubated and mechanically ventilated. Types of respiratory failures are listed further in the text. Providers should never delay intubation while

Table 5.1 Types of respiratory failure

Respiratory Failure (Type)	Mechanism
Type 1	Hypoxemia
Type 2	Hypercapnia
Type 3	Perioperative respiratory failure
Type 4	Detrimental WOB, Shock*

*The initiation of positive pressure ventilation is beneficial among patients with increased work of breathing due to the ability for positive pressure ventilation to decrease LV afterload, thereby improving cardiac output.[1]

awaiting blood gas analysis as this may delay care and result in emergency intubation. Upper airway obstructions such as laryngeal edema, vocal cord dysfunction, and pharyngeal abscess are also indications for intubation to prevent obstruction of the upper airway. Copious and/or thick bronchial secretions can require intubation for treatment and clearance to allow effective alveolar gas exchange. Patients who lack the ability to protect their airway should also be intubated. Typically, patients that can phonate have an adequate cough and swallow reflex and are able to protect their airway. A functioning swallow reflex is complex and involves the coordination of several oropharyngeal structures to prevent aspiration. In contrast, the absence of a gag reflex is less predictive of a patient's ability to protect their airway as up to 10% of the patient population may not have one.

Patients with brain injuries should be intubated for airway protection if there is a GCS ≤ 8, suspicion of impaired swallow/cough, concern for elevated ICP, impaired bronchial secretion clearance, apnea, or uncontrolled seizures. Alternatively, patients with high spinal cord injuries and peripheral neurologic disorders may also need to be intubated for impaired swallow/cough, impaired bronchial secretion clearance, and/or impending type 2 respiratory failure.

5.1.1.2   Airway Anatomy

Understanding airway anatomy is essential for airway management.
Mallampati grading is used to assess a patient's upper airway[2] as depicted
in Figure 5.1 and Table 5.2. This is done with the patient sitting upright and
sticking out their tongue.

5.1.1.3   Predictors of Difficult Mask Ventilation

Predictors of difficult mask ventilation among patients include BMI ≥ 26,
facial hair (beard), edentulous oral cavity, history of snoring, and age ≥55.[4]

Table 5.2 Mallampati grading of mouth aperture

Class	Description
Class I	Soft palate, uvula, tonsillar pillars visible
Class II	Uvula partially visible
Class III	Soft palate visible
Class IV	Unable to visualize soft palate

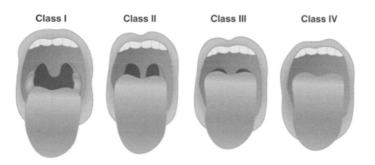

Figure 5.1 Mallampati grading depicting pharyngeal structures. Adapted from Miller's
Anesthesia Chapter 38.[3]

5.1.1.4 Predictors of Difficult Intubation

Predictors of difficult intubation include prior history, facial/airway trauma, and physical examination findings such as small mouth opening, Mallampati grade 3-4, inability for head and/or neck movement, mandible prominence/recession, large maxillary incisors, short thyromental distance, short sternomental distance, and obesity.[5]

5.1.1.5 Preoxygenation

Preoxygenation should occur whenever feasible. This should be performed with 100% oxygen with bag mask ventilation, HFNC, or NIPPV. One benefit of HFNC is that it can provide passive oxygenation during airway instrumentation.[6] Preoxygenation leads to denitrogenation of the alveoli, which provides an increased amount of time before desaturation occurs during apnea. Examples in which inadequate preoxygenation can occur are due to patient critical illness, high metabolic demand/minute ventilation, entrainment of room air secondary to poor mask seal, or the presence of a shunt.

5.1.1.6 Orotracheal Intubation

Direct laryngoscopy is typically performed with either a Miller or MacIntosh blade. The Cormack and Lehane grading scale[7] (Table 5.3) describes laryngoscopy views.

Table 5.3 Laryngoscopic views

Grade	Description
Grade 1	Entire glottic aperture visible
Grade 2	Posterior arytenoids visible, some of glottic aperture visible
Grade 3	Epiglottis visible
Grade 4	No visible structures

5.1.1.7   Confirmation of Intubation

Tracheal intubation should be confirmed by the presence of exhaled carbon dioxide via quantitative or colorimetric capnometry. Other markers of successful tracheal intubation include bilateral chest rise and water condensation within the endotracheal tube. Auscultation of the chest wall should be performed to rule out right mainstem intubation. As a generic rule, the orotracheal tube should be approximately 23 cm at the lip for males and 21 cm at the lip for females. Appropriate positioning can also be confirmed with a chest radiograph; the distal tip of the endotracheal tube should be 2–5 cm above the carina.

5.1.2   RAPID SEQUENCE INTUBATION

Rapid sequence intubation (RSI) should be considered for all patients who are suspected of having a high aspiration risk. Patients to consider include emergency cases, trauma patients, parturients, and patients with intraabdominal pathologies. The purpose of RSI is to minimize the time securing a patient's airway and to decrease the chance of aspiration.

Before the decision is made for RSI, the provider must balance the potential for difficulty in securing the airway against aspiration risk. Providers should have a well-established plan, including additional personnel and difficult airway equipment. In preparation for RSI, providers should avoid medications such as anxiolytics and analgesics as they may alter patient consciousness beyond the time required for intubation. Patients should be properly positioned. If time permits and the patient does not have any contraindications, the patient can be given non-particulate antacids, acid-suppressive medications, and prokinetics to decrease the risk of acid aspiration. Historically, the odds of developing aspiration pneumonitis, also known as Mendelson syndrome, occurs with aspiration of gastric contents with a pH <2.5 and volume >25 ml.

5.1.2.1　RSI Medications

A full review of the pharmacological agents used for induction is outside the scope of this chapter. A variety of medications can facilitate rapid sequence intubation and may include use of hypnotic, amnestic, analgesic, and paralytic agents with the goal of providing optimal intubating conditions.

Typical induction agents include etomidate, propofol, and ketamine. Etomidate has rapid onset/offset providing optimal intubating conditions with minimal impact on hemodynamics. Additional benefits include decreasing cerebral metabolic oxygen consumption. Among the downsides of etomidate use are myoclonus, the potential to develop adrenal insufficiency and inability to blunt the sympathetic stress response. Propofol is also a fast-acting compound with the benefit of rapid awakening as well as the ability to decrease cerebral metabolic oxygen consumption. Downsides of propofol use include hypotension due to myocardial depression and vasodilation, which can be detrimental when there is a need to preserve either cerebral or spinal perfusion pressure. Ketamine is a rapid acting medication that causes dissociative anesthesia with potential benefit of preservation of airway reflexes and respiratory drive. Additionally, ketamine can increase sympathetic tone. Disadvantages of ketamine use include increased cerebral metabolism as well as an increase in ICP due to an increase in cerebral blood flow.

The use of neuromuscular blocking agents is not always necessary, but it does facilitate intubation. Either depolarizing or non-depolarizing paralytic agents can be used. Succinylcholine has rapid onset/offset providing optimal intubating conditions in a short time period. It should be avoided in patients who have had an upregulation of extrajunctional nicotinic acetylcholine receptors (strokes, neuromuscular disorders, myopathies) as it can lead to hyperkalemic cardiac arrest. The use of high-dose rocuronium can also provide fast optimal intubating conditions; however, its duration is significantly longer than succinylcholine. If reversal of rocuronium is rapidly needed, sugammadex, a cyclodextrin, can quickly reverse rocuronium through molecular encapsulation.

5.1.2.2 Cricoid Pressure

Cricoid pressure, although controversial, can be applied to patients with high aspiration risk. It should be noted, however, that several studies have shown it to be ineffective and potentially harmful. When applied, cricoid pressure should be performed by an assistant and should be adjusted if the intubating provider has difficulty visualizing the airway.

5.1.2.3 Worst-Case Scenarios: Can't Intubate, Can't Ventilate

Despite proper assessment and planning, providers can still encounter difficult ventilation/intubation scenarios. Providers should be familiar with use of adjunct devices to intubate such as use of a tube introducer, videolaryngoscopes, and fiberoptic equipment. If continued difficulty is encountered, then temporization should occur with a supraglottic device such as a laryngeal mask airway (LMA). Certain LMAs allow for intubation through the device. A surgical airway is reserved as last resort.

5.1.2.4 Special Consideration for Brain Injuries (BIs)

Patients who have sustained a BI or suspected BI should be intubated with the goal of preventing further injury. Ideally, hypoxia and hypercapnia should be avoided, with an emphasis on maintaining hemodynamic stability. RSI should be performed. Patients with BI may have impaired autoregulation. Additional provider goals should be to optimize cerebral perfusion pressure (CPP). Medications used for induction must be titrated accordingly with an understanding of potential hemodynamic consequences. The use of neuromuscular blocking agents should be used to optimize intubating conditions. Additionally, providers must understand laryngoscopy is highly stimulating, potentially necessitating the use of short-acting antihypertensive agents such as esmolol or nicardipine. The use of ketamine in patients with BI has been questioned in the past, due to the concern for elevation of ICP, however, this has been unfounded. Additionally, use of a defasiculating medication before the use of succinylcholine in BI patients to prevent elevation of ICP is also unproven.

5.1.2.5   Special Consideration for Spinal Cord Injuries (SCIs)

The approach to airway management in patients who have sustained a SCI or suspected SCI depends on urgency, patient cooperation, difficulty of airway, and aspiration concerns. Up to 10% of TBI patients have SCI. These patients may present with immobilization devices making mask ventilation and intubation exceptionally challenging. Cervical spine motion during airway management should be avoided. Manual in-line stabilization (MIS) should be performed. If cricoid pressure is applied with a known cervical spine injury, it can potentially lead to further injury. When applied simultaneously, cricoid pressure and MIS can affect provider visualization and lead to increased intubation failure.

If the patient is cooperative and there is an allowance of time, providers may perform an awake intubation, especially if a difficult airway is suspected. Benefits of awake intubation include preservation of spontaneous ventilation, maintaining neutral head/neck, and immediate neurologic assessment post intubation. Patients who need emergency intubation should have an RSI with a videolaryngoscope with MIS to minimize cervical spine movement.

5.1.3   VENTILATOR MANAGEMENT

5.1.3.1   Basic Concepts

Invasive mechanical ventilation can fully or partially assist with work of breathing, allows for effective gas exchange, and can offset the metabolic demands during shock.[8] Typically, either volume or pressure parameters are chosen, depending on patient pathology and comorbidities.

For volume-controlled (VC) ventilation, the desired tidal volume (TV) to be reached with each breath is set. The pressure generated to deliver the TV is dependent on the set flow rate, pattern, and patient lung/chest wall compliance. Within VC ventilation, either assist-control (AC) or synchronized intermittent mechanical ventilation (SIMV) modes can be selected. When placed on AC-VC, a patient will receive the set TV during controlled breaths as well as when the patient triggers the ventilator. One benefit is that an AC-VC provides full ventilatory support and guarantees a set minute ventilation (MV). One downside of AC-VC is that it can lead to the development of respiratory alkalosis in patients with neurologic injury and respiratory center dysfunction further decreasing cerebral blood flow. Additionally, patients with obstructive lung disease can develop dynamic hyperinflation.

With SIMV-VC, the patient will receive a set TV with controlled breaths and allow for spontaneous breaths with or without pressure support. If the patient triggers the ventilator during SIMV-VC with a spontaneous breath before a controlled breath is delivered, the ventilator will synchronize with the patient's respiratory rate. A patient will receive the same MV with both AC-VC and SIMV-VC if the patient does not breathe faster than the set ventilator rate. While the use of SIMV-VC decreases the likelihood of developing respiratory alkalosis, it may also lead to a reduction of cardiac output and in some instances, in comparison to ACVC, can lead to an increase in work of breathing.

Pressure-controlled (PC) ventilation delivers a variable TV depending on pulmonary compliance. Recall that total airway pressure is inspiratory pressure plus PEEP. During PC ventilation, flow is delivered in a decelerating pattern until the pressure target is achieved. Like VC ventilation, either AC or SIMV modes can be selected with PC ventilation. By using PC ventilation, patients are less likely to develop volutrauma and barotrauma as the pressure target is set to a desired limit. In patients without pulmonary compliance issues, PC ventilation is well tolerated; however, providers should be aware of any changes in pulmonary compliance as a decrease can lead to underventilation.

BiLevel, also known as APRV, is PC mode of ventilation that allows spontaneous breaths and alternates between intermittent periods of high and low pressure. This mode of ventilation presumably benefits patients with lung injury[9] by preventing further damage and improving alveolar recruitment.

Pressure-regulated volume control (PRVC) is a pressure mode of ventilation. PRVC is available on new ventilators that allows a preset TV to be delivered with fluctuations in inspiratory flow. This mode of ventilation can lead to larger TV delivery than what is set due to variance in pulmonary compliance. Clinically, this mode has been found to have improved ventilator synchrony.

Pressure support (PS) ventilation is a spontaneous mode of ventilation that is typically used in weaning. As the patient triggers the ventilator, there is a set inspiratory pressure that is delivered above the PEEP. True pressure support does not have a back-up rate set. This can pose significant issues with pathologies that result in hypoventilation or apnea. Additionally, PS can be associated with increased WOB.

One goal of mechanical ventilation is to encourage active patient participation as early as possible. Persistent use of mechanical ventilation leads to muscle atrophy. No mode of ventilation has been proven to be superior to another. Generally, providers can interchange within VC and PC to generate similar MV. Irrespective of the mode of ventilation, patients should be monitored to ensure that adequate oxygenation/ventilation are achieved which can be assessed with clinical signs/symptoms and arterial blood gases.

5.1.3.2 Initiation of Mechanical Ventilation

An example for the initiation of VC ventilation include setting the respiratory rate (RR), tidal volume (TV), positive end expiratory pressure (PEEP), fractional inspired oxygen (FiO$_2$), and inspiratory flow. Common settings include a RR 10–14 per minute, TV 6–8 ml/PBW mL/kg of patient body weight, PEEP 5 cmH$_2$O, FiO$_2$ 40%, and inspiratory flow 60 l with a ramping pattern. It is critical that the patient be monitored, and ventilator settings be adjusted according to clinical scenario as well as blood gases.

5.1.3.3 Positive end Expiratory Pressure

PEEP improves oxygenation by recruiting alveoli and decreasing intrapulmonary shunting that may occur with atelectasis. Patients with BI may benefit from PEEP, especially to prevent hypoxemia. Providers should be aware of the potential risk for increased ICP as well decrease in MAP caused by high levels of PEEP.

5.1.3.4   Considerations for Acute Respiratory Distress Syndrome

Acute respiratory distress syndrome (ARDS) as defined by the Berlin criteria has significant morbidity and mortality. Ventilator strategy is to prevent further pulmonary insult. The ARDSnet protocol advocates for the use of lung-protective ventilation with low TVs with ideally 6 ml/kg PBW to achieve plateau pressures <30 cm H_2O. Oxygenation goals are either peripheral oxygen saturation target of >88% or PaO_2 goal >55 mmHg. Patients with BI can pose a challenge as tissue hypoxia can lead to secondary ischemic brain injury. Additionally, current ventilation strategies may lead to permissive hypercapnia, which can theoretically worsen brain injury; however, this is not currently still supported.[10]

5.1.3.5   Considerations for Brain Injury

Oxygenation goals for BI patients should be individualized. The Brain Trauma Foundation recommends targeting a PaO_2 >60 mmHg and peripheral O_2 saturation >90%.[11] Providers should also be aware that hyperoxia may cause cerebral vasoconstriction secondary to decreased cerebral blood flow (CBF).[12] Increased intrathoracic pressure during the inspiratory phase of mechanical ventilation can translate to decreased venous drainage and an increase in ICP, an effect that can be exacerbated by increased PEEP. However, PEEP should be used when clinically necessary and adjusted accordingly. Ventilation should be guided by blood gas, but $ETCO_2$ may also be used. Knowing the $ETCO_2$ to $PaCO_2$ gradient can be helpful, as $ETCO_2$ can be affected by variations in dead space. Hypercapnia should be avoided as it can increase CBF and worsen ICP. Hyperventilation can be used to acutely temporize patients with elevated ICP with a target $PaCO_2$ of 30–35 mmHg. However, these effects are diminished over time as bicarbonate levels within the extracellular fluid decrease and eventually lead to pH normalization (Figure 5.2). Excessive hyperventilation can lead to cerebral vasoconstriction and secondary ischemia from brain tissue hypoxia. There is also a theoretical risk with sudden return to eucapnia that can lead to a rebound increase in CBF and worsen ICP.

5.1.3.6 Sedation/Analgesia/Neuromuscular Blocking Agents During Mechanical Ventilation

A full review of the pharmacological agents used in the ICU is outside the scope of this chapter. Sedation is utilized in the ICU for numerous indications with an ideal RASS goal 0 to −2. Ideally nonbenzodiazepine agents should be used such as dexmedetomidine and propofol. Patient pain should be treated with analgesic agents such as fentanyl or hydromorphone. Neuromuscular block is infrequently used due to

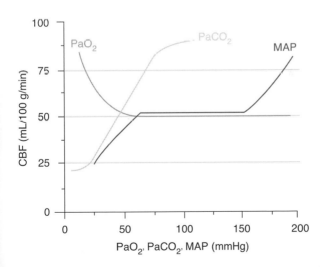

Figure 5.2 Alterations of cerebral blood flow. The effect of PaO_2 and $PaCO_2$ on CBF. Adapted from Miller's Anesthesia Chapter 17.[3]

potential disadvantages such as neuromuscular weakness and awareness due to inadequate sedation while paralyzed. Understanding the pharmacokinetics and pharmacodynamics of these agents is important. More so, understanding context-sensitive half-time is essential as these medications are given as infusions.

5.1.4 VENTILATOR DYSSYNCHRONY/ASYNCHRONY

Ventilator dyssynchrony or asynchrony typically occurs due to ventilator settings that do not adequately support the patient needs. This may lead to patient distress. Ventilator adjustments that may prevent/fix dyssynchrony include changing ventilator trigger, flow, and/or respiratory rate. If ventilator adjustments fail, one can consider increasing sedation and/or analgesia. As a last resort, neuromuscular blockade can be considered. Failure to correct ventilator dyssynchrony in patients with intracranial pathologies can lead to elevations in ICP due to transient increases in intrathoracic pressure.

5.1.4.1 Auto-PEEP

Auto-PEEP, also known as dynamic hyperinflation or "breath stacking," typically occurs in patients with obstructive lung disease. Patients are at increased risk for auto-PEEP with high minute ventilation. These patients may present with hemodynamic instability, respiratory distress, and eventually cardiac arrest. Examination of the flow time waveform on the ventilator will show that flow during expiration does not return to baseline. Expiratory breath hold may also reveal auto-PEEP. Strategies to prevent auto-PEEP include decreasing TV/RR, increasing expiratory time, and increasing inspiratory flow. Additionally, switching from AC ventilation to PS ventilation can also lead to improvement of auto-PEEP. If the occurrence of auto-PEEP is suspected during a situation where a patient has sudden hemodynamic instability the patient should immediately be disconnected from the ventilator to allow for passive exhalation.

Additionally, extrinsic compression of the chest can also lead to further lung deflation.

5.1.5 LIBERATION FROM MECHANICAL VENTILATION

Prolonged intubation and mechanical ventilation have been shown to increase the risk of ventilator-associated pneumonia (VAP), ventilator-induced lung injury (VILI), muscle atrophy, use of neuromuscular blockade agents, and increased use of sedatives. Patients who are intubated and mechanically ventilated should be assessed daily for discontinuation or liberation from mechanical ventilation. Providers can consider discontinuation of mechanical ventilation if patients exhibit cardiopulmonary stability and improvement or resolution of the pathology leading to intubation/mechanical ventilation. The liberation process can be either gradual or immediate with PSV/SIMV; however, spontaneous breathing trials (SBTs) with PSV are preferred.

Certain patients may be more difficult to liberate from mechanical ventilation due to cardiopulmonary pathologies, WOB, neurologic dysfunction, and metabolic derangements. These patients should still be assessed daily with spontaneous awakening trials (SATs) and SBTs.

5.1.5.1 Weaning/Extubation

The first step in vent weaning is to determine whether patients need full or partial ventilator support. Patients should be able to initiate spontaneous breaths and sustain the work of breathing with minimal, if any, mechanical support. Ideally, patients should only require a FiO_2 less than 40% and a PEEP less than 5–8 cmH$_2$O. Arterial oxygen saturation should be adequate. Blood gas analysis is not always needed, but if assessed it should reflect adequate ventilation and oxygenation. Patient readiness can be assessed clinically and with the use of the rapid shallow breathing index (RSBI). An RSBI greater than 105 breaths/min/L has been shown to be clinically predictive of weaning failure.[13] Weaning should occur with a daily SBT with PSV. An adequate

SBT trial should be at least 30 minutes and up to 120 minutes. SBT failure can consist of patient anxiety/agitation, increased WOB, RSBI > 105 breaths/min/L, hemodynamic instability and/or inefficient gas exchange. An additional assessment of lung mechanics should be performed with a vital capacity goal of >10 ml/kg[14] and negative inspiratory force (NIF) goal of <20 cmH$_2$O. VC requires full patient cooperation and is effort related. NIF indirectly assesses respiratory muscle strength.

The second step is determining any ongoing need for an artificial airway, which includes the assessment of a patient's ability to clear lower airway secretions. Thick and/or copious secretions may require treatments for secretion breakdown and deep suctioning and/or bronchoscopy for removal. Frequent suctioning of secretions, generally less than two hours, may prohibit removal of the artificial airway due to logistical challenges.

Third, upper airway obstruction can also lead to extubation failure. Removal of the artificial airway may lead to post-extubation stridor and potentially full obstruction of the upper airway. The determination of a cuff leak allows one to assess the presence or absence of airflow around a deflated endotracheal cuff. The presence of a cuff leak does not always ensure laryngeal patency and ability to participate in gas exchange, nor does the lack of a cuff leak indicate airway obstruction. In the appropriate clinical setting, the assessment of a cuff leak can provide insightful information including if the patient will be likely to develop post-extubation stridor. One can check a cuff leak using both quantitative and qualitative methods. Qualitative assessment includes deflation of the endotracheal cuff and audible assessment. Quantitative assessment is performed by assessing the difference in delivered and returned tidal volumes on mechanical ventilation.

If there is concern for a lack of cuff leak, several steps should be taken including elevation of the head of bed (HOB), diuresis if the patient is volume overloaded, and use of glucocorticoids for airway edema. Cuff leak can be reassessed every six to eight hours. Certain patients will never develop an adequate qualitative or quantitative cuff leak, as the selected endotracheal tube may be anatomically too large. Additionally, patients who have had recent surgery around the larynx/trachea (i.e. anterior cervical discectomy and fusion) may need time for resolution of inflammation and edema. Further assessment with either computed tomography or ultrasound can be considered to evaluate laryngeal obstruction. An attempt to extubate patients suspected of having laryngeal obstruction can occur with the understanding that they may need immediate reintubation. An airway assessment should be performed to determine if the re-intubation is likely to be challenging. Use of an airway exchange catheter (AEC) can be used to replace an endotracheal tube as a safety net. Additionally, an AEC can also be used for rescue ventilation/oxygenation until a more definitive airway can be established.

Fourth, a patient's level of consciousness should be assessed before extubation. Typically, an arousable, awake, or cooperative patient or a patient with a GCS of >8 has the ability for adequate airway protection.

5.1.5.2   CONSIDERATIONS FOR BRAIN INJURY

In general, patients with BI or strokes typically have higher rates of extubation failure due to altered level of consciousness, respiratory coordination, impaired, and/or inadequate coughing/swallowing. These patients typically do not have issues with lung mechanics, making classical assessment of extubation readiness insensitive. Numerous studies have attempted to offer further guidance assessing several parameters such as GCS, ability to follow simple commands, strength of cough, bronchial hygiene needs, and the presence of gag or cough, but none has consistently been able to consistently predict successful extubation. The VISAGE score is one such scoring system that has shown some promise in predicting extubation success if patients meet 3 of 4 criteria (visual pursuit,

swallowing, age <40 years, GCS >10).[15] Other studies have examined
a combination of viscosity of secretions, ability to follow four simple
commands.[16]

5.1.5.3 Considerations for Spinal Cord/Peripheral Neurologic Disorders

Patients with high spinal cord injuries and peripheral neurologic
disorders such as pathologies of the anterior horn, motor neuron, and
NMJ require an artificial airway and mechanical ventilation. These
patients may be unable to manage oropharyngeal as well as bronchial
secretions preventing extubation. Additionally, these patients typically
have chronic type 2 respiratory failure necessitating mechanical
ventilation. Lung mechanics must be thoroughly assessed (VC, NIF)
before consideration of liberation from mechanical ventilation.
Providers should consider early placement of tracheostomy if
prolonged artificial airway or mechanical ventilation is required.
These patients may benefit from therapies to assist in coughing as
well as secretion clearance.

5.1.5.4 High Risk of Reintubation

Patients who are at a high risk of reintubation should be closely
monitored. Many factors that have been found to increase risk include age
>65 years, COPD/pulmonary pathology, volume overload, prolonged
intubation, and need for emergency intubation. If there is concern for
oxygenation, one should consider extubating HFNC. Additionally, if there
is a concern for ventilation or cardiopulmonary dysfunction, one should
consider extubating to NIPPV. Patients who experience neuromuscular
dysfunction from myasthenia gravis[17] should be extubated to HFNC.
Provider vigilance is essential to detect impending respiratory failure,
which can present in various ways such as anxiety, sensation of increased
work of breathing and increased respiratory rate. For patients exhibiting
respiratory failure, the clinician should only trial either HFNC or NIPPV for

a short duration and reintubate to avoid further deterioration as delayed reintubation is associated with worse morbidity and mortality.

5.1.5.5 Tracheostomy

Patients admitted for neurologic pathologies or injuries exhibit higher tracheostomy rate of approximately 20–40% compared to the general critically ill population. Patients with neurologic injuries that cause an inhibition of respiratory drive and swallowing should be considered for tracheostomy. Moreover, patients with severe peripheral nerve disease and those with high cervical spine injuries should have a tracheostomy.[10] It is well established that tracheostomy provides several advantages including decreased chances of sinusitis, WOB, VAP, less sedation and increased ability for neurologic assessments. The decision on timing of tracheostomy is debatable; however, it should always be considered for patients who require an artificial airway, chronic respiratory failure, and/or those who fail weaning from mechanical ventilation. Early tracheostomy has proven beneficial in some patients, such as advanced ALS.

References

1. Pinsky MR. Cardiopulmonary interactions: physiologic basis and clinical applications. Ann Am Thorac Soc. 2018;15(Suppl 1):S45–48.
2. Samsoon GL, Young JR. Difficult tracheal intubation: a retrospective study. Anaesthesia. 1987;42(5):487–90.
3. Miller RD. Miller's anesthesia, 8th ed. Philadelphia, PA: Elsevier/Saunders; 2015, 2 vols., xxx, 3270, I–122.
4. Langeron O, Masso E, Huraux C, Guggiari M, Bianchi A, Coriat P, et al. Prediction of difficult mask ventilation. Anesthesiology. 2000;92(5):1229–36.
5. Apfelbaum JL, Hagberg CA, Caplan RA, Blitt CD, Connis RT, Nickinovich DG, et al. Practice guidelines for management of the difficult airway: an updated report by the American Society of Anesthesiologists Task Force on Management of the Difficult Airway. Anesthesiology. 2013;118(2):251–70.

6. Patel A, Nouraei SA. Transnasal Humidified Rapid-Insufflation Ventilatory Exchange (THRIVE): a physiological method of increasing apnoea time in patients with difficult airways. Anaesthesia. 2015;70(3):323–29.

7. Cormack RS, Lehane J. Difficult tracheal intubation in obstetrics. Anaesthesia. 1984;39 (11):1105–11.

8. Walter JM, Corbridge TC, Singer BD. Invasive mechanical ventilation. South Med J. 2018;111(12):746–53.

9. Zhou Y, Jin X, Lv Y, Wang P, Yang Y, Liang G, et al. Early application of airway pressure release ventilation may reduce the duration of mechanical ventilation in acute respiratory distress syndrome. Intensive Care Med. 2017;43(11):1648–59.

10. Chang WT, Nyquist PA. Strategies for the use of mechanical ventilation in the neurologic intensive care unit. Neurosurg Clin N Am. 2013;24(3):407–16.

11. Brain Trauma Foundation, American Association of Neurological Surgeons, Congress of Neurological Surgeons, Joint Section on Neurotrauma and Critical Care AANS/ CNS, Bratton SL, et al. Guidelines for the management of severe traumatic brain injury. I. Blood pressure and oxygenation. J Neurotrauma. 2007;24(Suppl 1):S7–13.

12. Floyd TF, Clark JM, Gelfand R, Detre JA, Ratcliffe S, Guvakov D, et al. Independent cerebral vasoconstrictive effects of hyperoxia and accompanying arterial hypocapnia at 1 ATA. J Appl Physiol. 2003;95(6):2453–61.

13. Yang KL, Tobin MJ. A prospective study of indexes predicting the outcome of trials of weaning from mechanical ventilation. N Engl J Med. 1991;324(21):1445–50.

14. Lermitte J, Garfield MJ. Weaning from mechanical ventilation. Cont Edu Anaesth Crit Care Pa. 2005;5(4):113–17.

15. Asehnoune K, Seguin P, Lasocki S, Roquilly A, Delater A, Gros A, et al. Extubation success prediction in a multicentric cohort of patients with severe brain injury. Anesthesiology. 2017;127(2):338–46.

16. Anderson CD, Bartscher JF, Scripko PD, Biffi A, Chase D, Guanci M, et al. Neurologic examination and extubation outcome in the neurocritical care unit. Neurocrit Care. 2011;15(3):490–97.

17. Rabinstein AA. Noninvasive ventilation for neuromuscular respiratory failure: when to use and when to avoid. Curr Opin Crit Care. 2016;22(2):94–99.

6

Neurocritical Care Pharmacology

Deepika P McConnell

Abstract

Patients in the neurological ICU can be challenging to care for, and treatment often involves complex medication regimens. This chapter provides a quick and concise reference to medication therapies used in the neurocritical care population. The topics span general critical care, including vasopressors and sedatives, but also provide guidance on treatment of neurospecific disease states such as sodium disorders and paroxysmal sympathetic hyperactivity, where robust data do not exist.

6.1 Hyperosmolar Agents

Hyperosmolar therapies are used widely among various neurological disease states such as intracranial hemorrhage (ICH), ischemic stroke, and traumatic brain injury (TBI). This treatment manages cerebral edema and may prevent cerebral herniation that can lead to brain death.

6.1.1 HYPEROSMOLAL TREATMENT

6.1.1.1 Hypertonic Saline (HTS)

HTS is available commercially or compounded in a wide variety of concentrations such as 2%, 3%, 7.5%, and 23.4% (Table 6.1). The most

Table 6.1 Hyperosmolar medications in the neurological ICU[1,2]

Drug	Mannitol 20%	Hypertonic saline 3%	Hypertonic saline 23.4%
Osmolarity	1098 mOsm/l	1025 mOsm/l	8008 mOsm/l
Dose	0.5–1.5 g/kg bolus and may repeat every 4–6 h	2.5–5 ml/kg bolus and/or 0.1–2 ml/kg/h continuous infusion	30 ml bolus
Administration	Bolus over 10–15 min Use 0.22 μm filter due to potential for crystallization May be administered through a peripheral line	Bolus over 10–15 min Central line preferred for infusion. If used peripherally, avoid prolonged administration	Bolus over 10 min MUST be given through CENTRAL line
Adverse effects	Acute renal failure Hypotension	Electrolyte abnormalities	Hypotension
Monitoring	Maintain serum Osm <320 and/or osmolar gap <20 mOsm/kg[2]	Serum sodium (Na) ~145–155	Serum sodium (Na)~145–155

common concentrations used are 3% and 23.4%. Both concentrations can be used as a bolus over 10–15 min in acute and emergent situations of elevated intracranial pressure (ICP) or cerebral herniation. Concentrations ≤3% may also be used as a continuous infusion to maintain serum sodium at goal and prevent further cerebral edema.

6.1.1.2 Mannitol

An osmotic diuretic is dosed based on actual body weight that reduces ICP by creating an osmotic gradient across the blood–brain barrier (BBB). The degree of ICP reduction achieved with mannitol is dose-dependent; therefore, doses ≥0.5 g/kg should be used.[1] Use cautiously in patients predisposed to acute renal failure (ARF), such as those with hypotension, sepsis, preexisting renal disease, and those on other nephrotoxic agents. The mechanism by which mannitol causes ARF is unclear, but it may be due to osmotic nephrosis, which is reversible with cessation of therapy or dialysis.[1]

Summary of Evidence-Based Literature

Overall, meta-analyses have shown a trend toward better ICP reduction with HTS versus mannitol. A meta-analysis done in 2015 showed that both mannitol and HTS reduce ICP but there is a trend toward greater ICP reduction with HTS. Results also showed that the duration of effect of HTS versus mannitol on ICP reduction was sustained for up to 120 min, suggesting a durable effect.[3] However, the clinical implications of the difference in ICP reductions remain unclear, and both agents are used effectively in clinical practice to treat intracranial hypertension in patients with TBI, ICH, SAH, ischemic stroke, and brain tumors.

6.2 Vasopressors

Vasopressor therapy is used in the neurocritical care (NCC) population for the treatment of hypotension related to shock and also, in select disease states, to induce hypertension (Tables 6.2 and 6.3). Selecting the appropriate vasopressor based on indication and patient characteristics is important. Vasopressors should be administered through a central line and used for the shortest duration at the lowest dose necessary to maintain adequate hemodynamics. Goals of therapy in the setting of hypotension are systolic blood pressure (SBP) ≥90 mmHg and/or mean arterial pressure (MAP) ≥65 mmHg measured by placement of continuous arterial blood pressure catheters.[4]

Table 6.2 Vasopressor comparison table[4,5]

Drug	Mechanism of action			Hemodynamic effects		
	Alpha-1	Beta-1	Beta-2	HR	SVR	CO
Norepinephrine (NE)	+++	++	0	↔/↑	↑↑	↔/↑
Phenylephrine	+++	0	0	↔/↓	↑	↓
Epinephrine	+++	+++	++	↑↑	↑	↑↑
Vasopressin	0	0	0	↔	↑	↓
Angiotensin II	0	0	0	↔/↑	↑↑	↓

HR = heart rate; SVR = systemic vascular resistance; CO = cardiac output

Summary of Evidence-Based Literature

Major randomized controlled trials (RCTs) and meta-analyses have shown higher mortality rates for the use of dopamine in various shock states compared to NE.[4] When compared to epinephrine in randomized studies, NE appears to have similar mortality rates. However, the incidence of adverse effects such as cardiac arrhythmias and lactic acidosis with epinephrine appears to be higher.[4] Therefore, NE is used as a first–line therapy for all major shock states in the ICU, including undifferentiated, vasodilatory, and hypovolemic shock.

Angiotensin II is the most recent addition to the vasopressor therapy arsenal. The ATHOS-3 study concluded that the use of angiotensin II in patients with vasodilatory shock, unresponsive to fluids and vasopressor therapy equivalent to NE 0.2 mcg/kg/min, increased MAP by 10 mmHg or to ≥75 mmHg in more patients than placebo without an increase in vasopressor doses. There was no difference in all-cause mortality at 7 or 28 days between placebo group and angiotensin II group.[6] Larger studies are necessary to determine long-term effects of angiotensin II and to detect mortality effects.

Table 6.3 Vasopressors in the ICU[4,5,6]

Drug	Dose	Adverse effects	Role in therapy
ADRENERGIC			
Norepinephrine	2–30 mcg/min	Tachyarrhythmias Tissue necrosis GI ischemia	First-line vasopressor in septic, cardiogenic, and hypovolemic shock[4]
Phenylephrine	50–300 mcg/min	Reflex bradycardia	Commonly used in the neurological ICU for induced hypertension for vasospasm and spinal cord perfusion Alternative vasopressor if patient has tachyarrhythmias
Epinephrine	2–10 mcg/min	Tachyarrhythmias Tissue necrosis GI ischemia	May be added to NE to meet MAP goals in refractory shock when HR and/or CO is low[4]
NON-ADRENERGIC			
Vasopressin	0.03–0.04 units/min (not titrated)	Cardiac and mesenteric ischemia Hyponatremia	May be added to NE as second line agent to meet MAP goals in refractory shock when HR is high and/or SVR is low[4] May be especially beneficial in acidemic patients
Angiotensin II	20 ng/kg/min and titrate by 15 ng/kg/min every 5 min to max 80 ng/kg/min in first 3 h and 40 ng/kg/min thereafter[6] As shock resolves down titrate by up to 15 ng/kg/min every 5–15 min[6]	Thromboembolism Delirium Lactic acidosis Tachycardia[5]	Should be reserved for salvage therapy in patients with septic shock May add on for vasodilatory shock unresponsive to fluids and vasopressors equivalent to NE 0.2 mcg/kg/min

6.3 Antihypertensives

Intravenous antihypertensives are a mainstay of treating hypertension in the neurological ICU given the need for rapid and aggressive blood pressure control in certain disease states (Table 6.4). Ideal antihypertensives are those with a quick onset and reliable dose response. Also important to consider are patient characteristics such as volume status, organ impairment, and heart rate when initiating antihypertensive therapy.

6.4 Sedatives (Table 6.5)

Some of the common indications for the use of sedatives in ICU include mechanical ventilation, elevated intracranial pressure, burst suppression for refractory status epilepticus, and adjunct to postoperative pain therapy. Critically ill patients may experience altered pharmacokinetics and pharmacodynamics due to impaired organ function, unstable hemodynamics, and fluid shifts altered protein binding and complex medication regimens leading to drug-drug interactions. These factors can lead to accumulation of sedatives and increased risk for adverse effects such as oversedation, hypotension, cardiac dysrhythmias, and metabolic disorders. Additionally, in the NCC patient, it is often difficult to assess whether an alteration in mental status is related to sedation or a change in the neurological exam associated with the injury. Therefore, individualized sedative titration as well as the use of sedation scales and nursing-driven sedation protocols or daily sedation interruptions is necessary to avoid excessive sedation and untoward effects.

Summary of Evidence-Based Literature

2018 SCCM PAD-IS guideline recommendations on sedation:

• Light sedation is preferred over deep sedation

Table 6.4 Antihypertensives in the neurological ICU[2,7]

Drug	Mechanism of action	Dose range	Onset	Duration	Adverse effects
Clevidipine (CI)	Calcium channel blocker	1–32 mg/h titrate every 90 s	2–4 min	5–15 min	Renal failure Headache Nausea
Enalaprilat (Intermittent)	ACE inhibitor	0.625 mg bolus, then 1.25–5 mg every 6 h	15–30 min	6 h	Headache Cough Profound hypotension
Esmolol (CI)	Cardioselective beta-blocker	0.5 mg/kg bolus then 50–300 mcg/kg/min	1–2 min	10–30 min	Bradycardia Nausea Bronchospasm
Hydralazine (Intermittent)	Arterial Vasodilator	10–20 mg IV every 4–6 h	5–10 min	1–4 h (can be up to 12 h)	Reflex tachycardia Headache Nausea
Labetalol (CI and intermittent)	Nonselective beta-blocker	Intermittent: 20–80 mg IV every 10 min CI: 0.5–2 mg/min Max: 300 mg/day	2–10 min	2–6 h	Orthostatic hypotension Nausea Bradycardia Bronchospasm
Nicardipine (CI)	Calcium channel blocker	CI: 2.5–15 mg/h Titrate by 2.5 mg every 15 min	5–15 min	30 min–4 h	Reflex tachycardia Headache Flushing Phlebitis

Medications in bold are most commonly used; CI = continuous infusions

Table 6.5 Sedatives in the ICU[2,8]

Drug	Mechanism of action	Dose	Adverse effects	Considerations
Dexmedetomidine	Alpha-2 agonist	CI: 0.2–1.5 mcg/kg/h Titrate by 0.1 mcg/kg/h every 10 min to sedation goal *loading doses are not recommended	Dose-related hypotension and bradycardia	No respiratory depression Provides some analgesic effects Titrate off if used >24 h due to potential for withdrawal effects
Lorazepam	GABA$_A$ receptor agonist	LD: 1–4 mg IV Intermittent dose: 1–4 mg every 2–6 prn CI: 0.5–8 mg/h Titrated to sedation goal	Hypotension Respiratory depression Delirium	Propylene glycol toxicity can occur at doses >1 mg/kg/day with prolonged infusion time. Toxicity is likely if osmolar gap >12 mmol/L with metabolic acidosis[9]
Midazolam	GABA$_A$ receptor agonist	LD: 0.5–4 mg every 15 min till sedation goal achieved CI: 2–5 mg/h Titrate to sedation goal Max: 0.1 mg/kg/h	Hypotension Respiratory depression Delirium	Caution in renal failure due to accumulation of active metabolites Prolonged infusions cause drug to accumulate in fat tissue CYP3A4 substrate
Propofol	GABA$_A$ receptor agonist	LD: 10–20 mg (only given to patients not hypotensive) CI: 5–50 mcg/kg/min Max: 67 mcg/kg/min Titrate every 5–10 min by 5–10 mcg/kg/min to sedation goal	Hypotension Apnea Hypertriglyceridemia Pancreatitis Propofol infusion syndrome (PRIS): severe metabolic acidosis, hyperkalemia, cardiac dysrhythmias and collapse rhabdomyolysis	Risk of PRIS is greatest in young patients, doses >67 mcg/kg/min and prolonged use >48 h.[2] Monitor CK, lactate, and TGs Dissolved in lipid emulsion delivering 1.1 kcal/ml

LD = loading dose

- Nursing-driven sedation or daily sedation interruptions may help maintain light levels of sedation
- Propofol or dexmedetomidine should be used over benzodiazepines
- Patients requiring a deep level of sedation for neuromuscular blockade or elevated intracranial pressure may benefit from the use of a bi-spectral index (BIS) monitor.

All of these recommendations appear to be ungraded or have a low quality of evidence. RCTs have not shown a significant benefit in terms of critical outcomes in patients on light versus deep sedation.[8] The lack of consensus on the definition of light, moderate, or deep sedation complicates the interpretation of these outcomes.

There are numerous studies investigating the difference in outcomes between the use of propofol or dexmedetomidine individually versus benzodiazepines. Overall, evidence shows a reduced time to light sedation and extubation but the differences were not clinically significant.[8]

6.5 Therapies for Sodium Disorders

Disorders of sodium such as syndrome of inappropriate antidiuretic hormone (SIADH), cerebral salt wasting syndrome (CSWS), and central diabetes insipidus (CDI) are frequent in the NCC population. If these conditions are left untreated, they can lead to serious complications such as cerebral edema, increased ICP, herniation, and possible death. It is important to note that the diagnosis of SIADH versus CSWS is challenging due to similar laboratory findings and careful clinical examination of volume status needs to be performed prior to initiation of treatment. Treatment strategies in Table 6.6 only include available pharmacological options but it should be noted that for each disease state, fluid management is usually the first-line therapy.

Table 6.6 Medications for sodium disorders in the neurological ICU[10,11]

Drug	Mechanism of action	Dose	Adverse effects	Clinical pearls
CDI				
Desmopressin (DDAVP)	Increases water resorption in the collecting tubule by agonizing renal V2 receptor	IV/SQ/IM: 0.5–2 mcg every 8–12 h Intranasal: 10–40 mcg/day (10 mcg = 1 spray) Oral: 50–600 mcg twice daily	Hyponatremia	Dose titrated based on urine output, serum sodium correction, and urine-specific gravity Whether patients need long-term therapy will depend on whether CDI is transient versus permanent or triphasic
SIADH				
Tolvaptan	V2 receptor antagonist	15–60 mg daily	Polydipsia polyuria diarrhea	Avoid use in patients with severe liver disease[10] Patients should drink fluids freely[11]
Conivaptan	V1A/V2 receptor antagonist	LD: 20 mg IVPB over 30 mins CI: 20–40 mg/day for maximum of 4 days	Phlebitis Orthostatic hypotension Hypokalemia	May be given peripherally Rotate site every 8–12 h to decrease risk of phlebitis May load daily without maintenance infusion and monitor sodium. This administration route may decrease risk of phlebitis[12]

Demeclocycline	Not well understood; increases water excretion by decreasing the responsiveness of the collecting tubule to ADH	300 mg oral twice daily May increase up to 1,200 mg/day	Nausea Vomiting Diarrhea Photosensitivity	Can take up to 1 week to see an effect
Sodium chloride tablets	Supplementation of sodium	4–16 g/day in 3 divided doses	Osmotic diarrhea	Data are limited
CSWS				
Fludrocortisone	Renal tubular reabsorption of sodium	100–600 mcg/day in 2–3 divided doses	Hypokalemia Hypertension	May develop tolerance if used >1 week

Summary of Evidence-Based Literature

The SALT studies investigated the effect of tolvaptan versus placebo in patients with euvolemic or hypervolemic hyponatremia in a mixed population in the outpatient setting. These studies found that in a majority of patients, tolvaptan effectively raised the sodium concentrations at 4 and 30 days of therapy.[10] Notably in these studies, patients with the lowest baseline sodium (severe hyponatremia) were those with the largest elevations of sodium with treatment; although none experienced osmotic demyelination. Therefore, if tolvaptan is being used in critically ill patients, careful sodium monitoring is crucial to avoid overcorrection.

One RCT evaluating intravenous conivaptan versus placebo in patients with euvolemic or hypervolemic hyponatremia found a greater increase in serum sodium and aquaresis in a larger number of patients on conivaptan. The study protocol included fluid restriction <2 L/day and loading dose of 20 mg followed by an infusion of 40 mg or 80 mg for 4 days.[10]

Outcome and comparison studies involving the use of V2 receptor antagonists for hyponatremia is lacking and therefore the role of these agents is reserved for refractory cases when other treatment modalities have been exhausted.

6.6 Alternative Routes of Drug Delivery

There are many factors that affect the entry of drugs into the central nervous system (CNS) such as molecular size, lipophilicity, protein binding, and active transport. Therefore, local administration of medications through the intrathecal/intraventricular and intra-arterial route are available options to overcome the difficulty of penetrating the BBB. It is important to note that the evidence for the use of medications through these routes is not robust and the recommendations for dosing regimens, concentrations, and duration originate mainly from retrospective case series and cohort studies. As a result, these routes are usually reserved for cases refractory to conventional medication therapy.

6.6.1 INTRA-ARTERIAL

Intra-arterial administration is reserved for administration of medications intra-procedurally through a catheter, at the site of lesion or vasospasm, by an interventional neuroradiologist or neurosurgeon (Table 6.7). Indications include cerebral vasospasm after aneurysmal subarachnoid hemorrhage refractory to conventional medical therapy and also in acute ischemic stroke when intravenous thrombolytics have failed or if the patient is not a candidate to receive intravenous thrombolytic therapy.

Table 6.7 Intra-arterial (IA) medications

Drug	Dose	Special considerations
Alteplase	<20 mg[13]	Administered in dosing aliquots until thrombus is resolved
		Usually given in conjunction with mechanical thrombectomy
Nicardipine	10–40 mg per vessel[14]	First line for treatment of refractory vasospasm[14]
Verapamil	2.5–360 mg per vessel[14]	May cause mild and transient ICP elevation and systemic hypotension[14]
Milrinone	5–24 mg[14]	May have a role for patients not tolerant of IA nicardipine[14]
		Usually followed by treatment with IV milrinone in available studies
		Potential for rebound vasospasm

Table 6.8 Treatment options for ITB withdrawal[15–17]

Drug	Dose	Special considerations
Oral baclofen	10–20 mg every 6 h	Slow onset of action and time to peak effect
	Dose increased to >120 mg/day in divided doses	Does not readily cross BBB
		Alternative agents or ITB bolus dosing should be used for early acute withdrawal in addition to oral baclofen[15]
Lorazepam or Midazolam	1–2 mg every 2–4 h Titrate to effect	Initiate IV therapy and transition to oral
		Rapid titration may be necessary to achieve muscle relaxation, normothermia, and hemodynamic stabilization[15]
Diazepam	2.5–5 mg every 6–8 h Titrate to effect	Same as above
Cyproheptadine	4–8 mg every 6–8 h	Use as adjunct for reduction in tone and spastic hypertonia. May also alleviate other symptoms such as itching and fever[16]
Tizanidine	8–12 mg in 3–4 divided doses	Use as adjunct for acute increase in spasticity and tone[15]
Dantrolene	Varies widely Oral: 12.5 mg bid IV: 2.5–10 mg/kg in divided doses	Use as adjunct for extreme muscle spasticity refractory to other therapies[17]
Intrathecal baclofen	Bolus: 50 mcg	**Only done by ITB physician expert:** Infusion or bolus may be administered through placement of external intrathecal catheter. Bolus may be also given through access port on pump if catheter is connected or lumbar puncture[15]
	Maintenance infusion: 12–2003 mcg/day or similar dose as before therapy was interrupted	Avoided in patients with infectious concern

Table 6.9 Opioid conversion table

Drug	Intrathecal (mg)	Intravenous (mg)	Oral (mg)
Morphine	1	200	300
Hydromorphone	0.2	20	60
Fentanyl	0.01	1	—

Reproduced with permission from: Cohen and Dragovich[18]

6.6.2 INTRATHECAL

Intrathecal drugs are delivered directly into the lumbar cistern through temporary catheter or long term subcutaneous implanted pump. Medications commonly administered through this route include opiates like morphine and hydromorphone, as well as baclofen for intractable spasticity.

Most ICU admissions for patients with intrathecal pumps are due to pump failures or the need for pump removal due to an infection. These conditions cause abrupt discontinuation of the medication leading to high risk for medication withdrawal. In order to mitigate withdrawal and life-threatening complications replacement therapy is necessary. Tables 6.8 and 6.9 provide alternative therapy for intrathecal baclofen (ITB) and opiates in the setting of abrupt discontinuation.

6.6.3 INTRAVENTRICULAR (TABLE 6.10)

The administration of medications such as antibiotics, chemotherapy, and thrombolytics directly into the lateral ventricle to overcome the BBB by either ventriculostomy or reservoir. Drug delivery by this route allows higher concentrations of medication in the cerebrospinal fluid (CSF) compared to when given intravenously.

Table 6.10 Intraventricular medications[19-22]

Drug	Dose	Diluent/volume antimicrobials	Special considerations
Colistin	10 mg	Diluent: 0.9% normal saline (NS) Final volume: 3 ml	Reserve use for CNS infections caused by multi-drug-resistant (MDR) gram-negative bacteria
Polymyxin B	5 mg	Diluent: 0.9% NS Final volume: 3 ml	
Amikacin	30 mg Dose range: 5–50 mg	Diluent: 0.9% NS Final concentration: 30 mg/ml	Amikacin is not available in a preservative-free (PF) formulation Use PF gentamicin and tobramycin
Gentamicin	4–8 mg	Diluent: 0.9% NS Final concentration: 2 or 5 mg/ml	Adverse effects not well reported in literature but monitor for seizures, hearing loss, and aseptic meningitis[19]
Tobramycin	5–10 mg	Diluent: 0.9% NS Final concentration: 5 mg/ml	
Vancomycin	10–20 mg	Diluent: 0.9% NS Final concentration: 2.5, 5 or 10 mg/ml depending on dose	No serious toxicities have yet been reported[20]
Daptomycin	5–10 mg	Diluent: 0.9% normal saline (NS) Final volume: 3 ml	May dose daily for first 2–3 days and then every 72 h[21] Used in patients with MDR gram-positive bacteria, such as vancomycin-resistant enterococcus or staphylococcus epidermidis
Amphotericin B deoxycholate	0.01–0.5 mg	Diluent: 5% dextrose in water Final volume: 2 ml	Used in patients with Candida shunt infections who fail systemic therapy or shunt removal[21]
Vasodilators			
Nicardipine	2–4 mg every 8–12 h	Diluent: 0.9% NS Final volume: 2 ml	First-line therapy for refractory vasospasm in SAH
Thrombolytics			
Alteplase	1 mg every 8 h	Diluent: sterile water Final volume: 1 ml	Not routinely recommended for intraventricular hemorrhage[22]

6.6.3.1 Clinical Pearls for Intraventricular (IVT) Medications[19–21]

- Ensure that medication and diluent used are preservative free when possible.
- Instillation of intraventricular medication should be administered by trained staff.
- When medication is administered through an external ventricular drain (EVD), the drain should be clamped for 15–60 min to allow for equilibration of drug.
- The evidence for use of CSF therapeutic drug monitoring (TDM) for IVT antimicrobial therapy is unclear. Selective TDM may be useful when dose is outside of the usual range, CSF cultures are persistently positive, patients remain symptomatic, toxicity is suspected, duration of therapy is extended, or when there are changes to CSF production, flow, and clearance. A limitation in obtaining CSF drug concentrations is whether the laboratory is able to provide results in real time and with a rapid turnaround time. Also, the therapeutic range available in the literature is wide and not well established.
- Per IDSA guidelines, IVT vancomycin and gentamicin dosing varies based on ventricular size and volume. Also recommended is to adjust frequency of dosing based on EVD output.

6.7 Paroxysmal Sympathetic Hyperactivity (PSH, Table 6.11)

A significant percentage of patients with acquired brain injury will develop autonomic dysfunction presenting with a constellation of symptoms such as fevers, tachycardia, tachypnea, hypertension, diaphoresis, and dystonia. Treatment of these symptoms is important to prevent end organ dysfunction.[23] There is a wide variety of pharmacologic options for prevention and symptomatic treatment, although application of these medications is not based on randomized controlled clinical trials.

Table 6.11 Treatment options for paroxysmal sympathetic hyperactivity

Drug	Dose	Indication	Adverse effects	Clinical pearls
Dexmedetomidine	CI: 0.2–1.5 mcg/kg/h *Do not use LD	Hypertension Agitation Tachycardia	Hypotension Bradycardia	Used in ICU setting Transition to oral clonidine when stable
Morphine	1–2 mg every 1–2 h prm	Tachycardia Peripheral vasodilation Allodynia	Respiratory depression Sedation	Therapeutic effect is rapid and dose-dependent May need to transition to oral opiates when stable
Lorazepam	2–4 mg IV every 2–4h prm	Agitation Hypertension Tachycardia Posturing	Respiratory depression Sedation	Used for breakthrough episodes Convert to clonazepam to prevent hyperactivity and withdrawal
Midazolam	1–2 mg IV every 2h prm	Agitation Hypertension Tachycardia Posturing	Respiratory depression Sedation	Used for breakthrough episodes Convert to clonazepam to prevent hyperactivity and withdrawal
Diazepam	1–10 mg IV every 4h prm	Agitation Hypertension Tachycardia Posturing	Respiratory depression Sedation	Used for breakthrough episodes Convert to clonazepam to prevent hyperactivity and withdrawal
Clonazepam	0.5–8 mg PO in 3 divided doses	Agitation Hypertension Tachycardia Posturing	Respiratory depression Sedation	Used for preventive therapy

Drug	Dose	Indications	Side effects	Comments
Clonidine	0.1–0.3 mg PO TID Max: 1.2 mg/day	Hypertension Tachycardia	Hypotension Bradycardia	Careful titration to avoid hypotension in between PSH episodes[23] Avoid abrupt discontinuation as this can result in rebound hypertension
Propranolol	20–60 mg PO every 4–6h	Hypertension Tachycardia Fever	Hypotension Bradycardia Bronchospasm	Highly lipophilic and penetrates BBB Careful titration to avoid hypotension in between PSH episodes[23]
Gabapentin	100–300 mg PO TID Max: 4800 mg/day	Allodynia Spasticity	Sedation	Well tolerated
Bromocriptine	1.25 mg PO BID Titrate to 40 mg/day	Dystonia Posturing Fever Diaphoresis	Nausea Confusion Agitation Dyskinesias	May lower seizure threshold Delayed therapeutic effect[23]
Baclofen	5 mg PO TID Max: 80 mg/day	Pain Clonus Rigidity	Sedation	Avoid abrupt discontinuation due to potential for withdrawal
Dantrolene	0.25–2 mg/kg IV every 6–12 h Max: 10 mg/kg/day	Severe dystonic posturing Muscle rigidity	Hepatotoxicity Respiratory depression	Avoid in patients with hepatic disease Monitor LFTs

Adapted with permission from: Thomas and Greenwald[24]

6.8 Utilizing the Clinical Pharmacist (Tables 6.12 and 6.13)

Table 6.12 What does a neurocritical care pharmacist do?

Medication profile review	Review patient's medications to determine safety and efficacy.
Assist in making pharmacotherapy decisions	Select appropriate antihypertensive, sedative, antibiotic, anti-epileptic and any other medication based on organ function, drug-drug interactions, co-morbid conditions, cultures and site of infection, allergies etc.
Therapeutic drug monitoring	Interpret and adjust doses of medications such as vancomycin, aminoglycosides, digoxin, phenytoin, phenobarbital, and valproic acid based on serum drug concentrations, goal therapeutic levels, and clinical goals. **Don't treat the number, treat the patient.**
Drug information	Perform literature searches to critically evaluate all levels of data available in order to provide appropriate treatment options.
Emergency response	Respond to cardiac arrests. Critical care pharmacists assist by providing drug information, calculating doses and infusion rates, preparing medications at the bedside, and setting up pump devices. Some institutions also include pharmacist response to emergent airway placements, stroke, and ICH codes to assist in medication management.
Medication reconciliation	Obtain the most accurate home medication list and assist in determining what medications are appropriate to be resumed.
Patient and family education	Provide medication counseling to patients identified to be on new medications or noncompliant with medication regimens.

Table 6.13 How to best use your critical care pharmacist

Communication	Notify your pharmacist prior to a new patient transfer who may need emergent pharmacological intervention.
	Involve your pharmacist early in interventions for a deteriorating patient to help prevent the situation from escalating. The pharmacist can quickly get medications to the bedside.
	When placing an order for a medication and are uncertain of the dose, route, frequency, etc., contact your pharmacist for the correct information prior to placing the order.
Utilization	Don't be afraid to ask for help at any time before, during or after rounds – this is the pharmacist's role and they are happy to be involved in all aspects of patient care.
	Prior to changing antibiotics based on new culture results, ask your pharmacist for assistance. Pharmacists can provide insight into the hospital's antibiogram and MIC of the organism or other patient specific factors, which are essential information to consider when switching antibiotics
	When drug serum concentrations result, consult your pharmacist for assistance on adjusting medication doses. Factors such as timing, measurement technique, drug–drug interactions, and patient specific considerations such as dialysis or renal replacement therapy and protein binding can affect accurate interpretation of the results.
Education	Ask your pharmacist to provide educational sessions or lectures for new trainees or refreshers for seasoned staff. Clinical pharmacists can impart knowledge about new medications, the latest research, or provide general information about pharmacological management on any disease state.
Collaboration	Interdisciplinary teams are successful teams and provide the best patient care. At our institution, pharmacists are involved in a variety of committees, research, and conferences with physician staff, which helps elevate our practice as well as yours.

References

1. Torre-Healy A, Marko NF, Weil RJ. Hyperosmolar therapy for intracranial hypertension. Neurocrit Care. 2012;17:117–30.

2. Brophy GM, Human T. Pharmacotherapy pearls for emergency neurological life support. Neurocrit Care. 2017;27:51–73.

3. Li M, Chen T, Chen S, et al. Comparison of equimolar doses of mannitol and hypertonic saline for the treatment of elevated intracranial pressure after traumatic brain injury: a systematic review and meta-analysis. Medicine. 2015;94(17):e736.

4. Jentzer JC, Coons JC, Link CB, Schmidhofer M. Pharmacotherapy update on the use of vasopressors and inotropes in the intensive care unit. J Cardiovasc Pharmacol Ther. 2015;20(3):249–60.

5. Bauer SR, Sacha GL, Lam SW. Safe use of vasopressin and angiotensin II for patients with circulatory shock. Pharmacotherapy. 2018;38(8):851–61.

6. Khanna A, English S, Wang XS, et al. Angiotensin II for the treatment of vasodilatory shock. N Engl J Med. 2017;377:419–30.

7. Rose JC, Mayer, SA. Optimizing blood pressure in neurological emergencies. Neurocrit Care. 2004;1:287–99.

8. Devlin JW, Skrobik Y, Gélinas C, et al. Clinical practice guidelines for the prevention and management of pain, agitation/sedation, delirium, immobility, and sleep disruption in adult patients in the ICU. Crit Care Med. 2018;46(9):e825-73.

9. Yahwak JA, Riker RR, Fraser GL, Subak-Sharpe S. Determination of a lorazepam dose threshold for using the osmol gap to monitor for propylene glycol toxicity. Pharmacotherapy. 2008;28(8):984–91.

10. Buffington MA, Abreo K. Hyponatremia: a review. Intensive Care Med. 2016;31 (4):223–36.

11. Chester KW, Rabinovich M, Luepke KH, et al. Sodium disorders in critically ill neurologic patients: a focus on pharmacologic management. OA Crit Care. 2014;2(1):2.

12. Murphy T, Dhar R, Diringer M. Conivaptan bolus dosing for the correction of hyponatremia in the neurointensive care unit. Neurocrit Care. 2009;11(1):14–19.

13. Castonguay AC, Jumaa MA, Zaidat OO, et al. Insights into intra-arterial thrombolysis in the modern era of mechanical thrombectomy. Front Neurol. 2019;10:1195.

14. Dabus G, Nogueira RG. Current options for the management of aneurysmal subarachnoid hemorrhage-induced cerebral vasospasm: a comprehensive review of the literature. Interv Neurol. 2013;2(1):30–51.

15. Ross JC, Cook AM, Stewart GL, et al. Acute intrathecal baclofen withdrawal: a brief review of treatment options. Neurocrit Care. 2011;14:103–08.

16. Meythaler JM, Roper JF, Brunner RC. Cyproheptadine for intrathecal baclofen withdrawal. Arch Phys Med Rehabil. 2003;84(5):638–42.

17. Coffey RJ, Edgar TS, Francisco GE, et al. Abrupt withdrawal from intrathecal baclofen: recognition and management of a potentially life-threatening syndrome. Arch Phys Med Rehabil. 2002;83:735–41.

18. Cohen SP, Dragovich A. Intrathecal analgesia. Anesthesiol Clin. 2007;25(4):863–82. Table 1, Conversion ratios between commonly used opioid agonists; p 865.

19. LeBras M, Chow I, Mabasa VH, et al. Systematic review of efficacy, pharmacokinetics, and administration of intraventricular aminoglycosides in adults. Neurocrit Care. 2016;25(3):492–507.

20. Ng K, Mabasa VH, Chow I, et al. Systematic review of efficacy, pharmacokinetics, and administration of intraventricular vancomycin in adults. Neurocrit Care. 2014;20:158–71.

21. Tunkel AR, Hasbun R, Bhimraj A, et al. 2017 Infectious Diseases Society of America's clinical practice guidelines for healthcare-associated ventriculitis and meningitis. Clin Infect Dis. 2017;64(6):e34–65.

22. Kiser, TH. Cerebral vasospasm in critically ill patients with aneurysmal subarachnoid hemorrhage: does the evidence support the ever-growing list of potential pharmacotherapy interventions? Hosp Pharm. 2014;49:923–41.

23. Rabinstein AA, Benarroch EE. Treatment of paroxysmal sympathetic hyperactivity. Curr Treat Options Neurol. 2008;10:151–57.

24. Thomas A, Greenwald BD. Paroxysmal sympathetic hyperactivity and clinical considerations for patients with acquired brain injuries: a narrative review. Am J Phys Med Rehabil. 2019;98(1):65–72. Table 4, Pharmacologic options for the treatment of PSH; p 69.

7

Intracerebral Hemorrhage

Brandon Francis

Abstract

Intracerebral hemorrhage (ICH) is spontaneous bleeding within the
brain parenchyma. ICH only represents about 20% of all strokes but
is disproportionately morbid. Most ICH patients present with an
acute neurologic deficit that can be differentiated from ischemic
stroke with a computed tomography scan. Rapid clinical assessment, blood pressure control, and reversal of coagulopathy are the
hallmarks of acute ICH management. It is important to monitor for
and treat complications such as intraventricular hemorrhage, cerebral edema, and seizures. Outcomes can be communicated by
functional assessments but it is optimal to include quality of life
information that matter to patients and caregivers.

7.1 Definition and Epidemiology

Intracerebral hemorrhage (ICH) is a subtype of stroke that refers to
spontaneous bleeding into the brain parenchyma[1,2] (this chapter does not
address traumatic ICH). It accounts for up to 15% of all strokes in the
United States and up to 27% of all strokes worldwide.[1,3] ICH
disproportionately impacts morbidity and mortality and can exceed 50%
at one year.[3,4] Importantly, rapid stabilization, assessment, and
management can impact morbidity and mortality.[1,4]

7.2 Initial Assessment and Management

7.2.1 CLINICAL EXAM

The clinical exam is the most important part of acute care for any patient, and those with acute neurologic injury are no exception. Your initial evaluation will give insights into the diagnostic and therapeutic interventions required. As with all patients, obtaining a brief history may be helpful in determining last known normal, comorbidities, and likely contributing factors such as therapeutic anticoagulation.

Clinically, the most common presentation of ICH is acute onset of a new neurologic deficit similar to acute ischemic stroke.[1,2,5] ICH patients more commonly present with markedly elevated blood pressure, abnormal consciousness, headache, and vomiting.[5] However, it is difficult to reliably distinguish between ICH and acute ischemic stroke without appropriate neuroimaging.[2,5]

7.3 Stabilize the Patient

It is paramount to ensure that the patient is stable. Frequent and repeated assessments of the patient's airway, breathing, and circulation are critical. Many comatose patients, who can be conceptualized as patients with a Glasgow Coma Score (GCS) of <8, may benefit from invasive mechanical ventilator support. This is because many comatose patients may have limitations in the ability to perform adequate gas exchange, address metabolic abnormalities, and protect their airway. A reasonable initial ventilatory target is eucapnia.[2]

Patients with ICH can also have hemodynamic abnormalities. Many patients will present with hypertension but some may be hypotensive and may require fluid resuscitation to ensure adequate intravascular volume.[2]

7.4 Neuroimaging

Emergent, noncontrast computed tomography (CT) scans are the most common initial neuroimaging modality used in the diagnosis of ICH. CT examinations can be obtained in a few moments, have high sensitivity and specificity for ICH and can accommodate patients with a wide variety of supportive devices. Magnetic resonance imaging (MRI) can also be used to diagnose ICH; however, costs, logistics of accessing the study, and required supportive devices may limit its use.[1,2]

Neuroimaging can offer insights into the etiology of the ICH. Locations such as the basal ganglia, brain stem, and cerebellum are more commonly related to hypertension. Lobar locations often are related to amyloid angiopathy or arteriovenous malformations.[2,5]

Hematoma expansion, which occurs in up to 40% of patients, is a strong predictor of outcome in ICH.[1,2] The volume of the ICH can be estimated using the ABC/2 formula, which approximates the volume of an ellipse.[6] Repeated non-contrast CT imaging at an appropriate interval and initial CT angiography (CTA) imaging can be considered to evaluate for hematoma expansion.[2,5] The "spot sign" that describes extravasated contrast within a hematoma may indicate ongoing hematoma growth.[2,7]

7.5 Blood Pressure Targets

The 2015 American Heart Association/American Stroke Association (AHA/ASA) guidelines indicate that for ICH patients with an initial systolic blood pressure (SBP) between 150 and 220 mmHg targeting a systolic blood pressure of 140 mmHg is safe.[1] This was largely based on the results and interpretation of the Intensive Blood Pressure in Acute Cerebral Hemorrhage (INTERACT2) trial. The INTERACT2 trial evaluated 2,794 ICH patients and compared early (within 1 h of presentation) intensive blood pressure control (<140 mmHg) to standard care at the time

(<180 mmHg). The study demonstrated that 52% (719 of 1,382) in the intensive group (SBP <140 mmHg) compared to 55.6% (785 of 1,412) of usual care (SBP <180 mmHg) had achieved the primary outcome of a Modified Rankin Score (mRS) of ≥3 (death or disability; OR 0.87; 95% CI, 0.75–1.01; P = 0.06). Ordinal analysis of the mRS demonstrated OR 0.87; 95% CI, 0.77–1.00; P = 0.04. It should be noted that intensive early blood pressure control did not seem to significantly impact hematoma expansion.[1,8]

The optimal blood pressure target has come into question with more recent data. The Antihypertensive Treatment of Acute Cerebral Hemorrhage (ATACH2) trial evaluated 1,000 patients and compared SBP 110–139 mmHg to 140–179 mmHg within 4.5 h of symptom onset. There was no difference in mortality or hematoma expansion between the two groups. However, a statistically significant increase in neurological deterioration within the first 24 h was observed in the intensive (SBP <140 mmHg) group (10.4%; aRR, 1.98;95% CI, 1;.08–3.62) and in a group that was initially reduced but was unable to maintain that lower blood pressure target (11.5%; aRR, 2.08; 95% CI, 1.15–3.75). There was also an increase (although, not statistically significant) in both renal and cardiac-related adverse events. These negative effects seemed to be independent of whether or not the lower blood pressure target (SBP <140 mmHg) was able to be maintained for the duration of the study period.[9,10]

This presents a challenging situation. The guidelines have not been updated since 2015 to reflect the synthesis of and an expert consensus approach to more recent data. The Neurocritical Care Society (NCS), the professional society of neurointensivists and professionals in the field of neurocritical care, suggests it is reasonable to target SBP 140–180 mmHg. Blood pressure control should occur rapidly and with an agent that can be administered intravenously, has a quick onset of action, and allows for titration. Examples of intravenous agents include labaetalol, clividipine, enalaprilat, and nicardipine.[2]

7.6 Reversal of Coagulopathies

Coagulopathy in ICH can increase the size of the initial hematoma, increase the risk of hematoma expansion, and can lead to increased mortality. There are a variety of etiologies for coagulopathy from neoplastic disease to hepatic failure to different classes of pharmacologic agents.[1,2,5]

Patients with coagulopathy related to vitamin K antagonists (e.g. warfarin) should receive prothrombin complex concentrates (PCC). Traditionally, fresh frozen plasma (FFP) has been used to reverse the coagulopathy. While effective, FFP takes longer to achieve hemostasis and has an increased risk of complications including logistical limitations (e.g. has to be thawed prior to use), transfusion-related reactions, and pulmonary edema. The target INR should be ≤1.4 and while no specific INR target has been prospectively determined for external ventricular drain (EVD) placement, ≤1.5 is typically considered safe.[2]

Antiplatelet agents, such as aspirin or clopidogrel, may also increase the risk of hematoma expansion. To address abnormal platelet function, some centers use specific platelet function testing while others empirically transfuse platelets.[2] In 2016, the PATCH (platelet transfusion versus standard care after acute stroke due to spontaneous cerebral hemorrhage associated with antiplatelet therapy) evaluated 190 patients with ICH who were also on antiplatelet therapy. Patients who required neurosurgical intervention were excluded. The authors found increased rates of disability or death in the transfusion group (OR 2.05, 95% CI 1.18–3.56; $P = 0.01$) without significant improvement in hematoma growth.[11] Consequently, the NCS only recommends platelet transfusion for patients on antiplatelet agents if they require neurosurgery.[2] It is reasonable to consider a single dose of desmopressin to reverse pharmacologic antiplatelet effect.[2,12] AHA/ASA guidelines to recommend platelet transfusion for severe thromocyopenia.[1]

Direct thrombin inhibitors and factor Xa inhibitors can also cause life-threatening coagulopathy in the setting of ICH and have targeted reversal agents. Direct thrombin inhibitors (e.g. dabigatran) can be reversed with idarucizumab, a monoclonal antibody, and is recommended for patients with ICH on dabigatran. Factor Xa inhibitors (e.g. rivaroxaban) can be reversed with adnexanet alpha. While it is expensive and may have some prothrombotic effects, it is currently recommended by the NCS to reverse factor Xa inhibitor coagulopathy in patients with ICH. If a targeted reversal agent is not available, it is possible to use prothrombin complex concentrates (4-factor and factor VIII inhibitor bypass activity); however, they do not demonstrate full coagulopathy reversal and have not been evaluated in multiple prospective, randomized controlled trials. FFP is of unclear benefit in patients with direct thrombin inhibitor or factor Xa inhibitor coagulopathy and ICH.[2]

Low-molecular-weight heparin and unfractionated heparin can be targeted for reversal with protamine sulfate. It should be noted that protamine sulfate only incompletely reverses low-molecular-weight heparin.[1]

7.7 Scoring Systems

The National Institute of Health Stroke Scale (NIHSS) may not always be helpful in communicating severity of illness and risk of mortality in ICH. Clinical and imaging characteristics (e.g. hematoma location) that have been shown to correlate with disease severity are not captured by the NIHSS.[1]

The Intracerebral Hemorrhage Score is required documentation by the Joint Commission for patients with ICH. The ICH score indicates severity of illness and is scored from zero (low expected mortality, lowest severity) to six (likely death, highest severity). It accounts for clinical and imaging characteristics that closely correlate to mortality.[1,2,5]

7.8 Neurosurgical Intervention

It has been postulated that early neurosurgical hematoma evacuation would improve outcomes. Surgical hematoma evacuation addresses important pathophysiologic concepts such as the removal of cytotoxic blood degradation products, decreased risk of hematoma-associated herniation, and decreased risk of dangerous intracranial pressure elevations.[2] Several important surgical trials evaluating outcomes in patients with hematoma evacuation provide much of the data and inform our understanding regarding potential roles for neurosurgical intervention in patients with ICH.

STICH I evaluated 1,033 patients of which 468 were randomized to early surgery. At a prespecified 6-month time point, 122 (26%) compared to 118 (24%) of 496 had a favorable outcome as determined by the mRS and the Extended Glasgow Outcome Scale (OR 0.89; 95% CI 0.66–1.19; $P = 0.4$). STICH I demonstrated no harm from the procedure, but no mortality benefit. Upon subgroup analysis, it appeared that lobar hematoma evacuation may confer a benefit.[13]

STICH II evaluated lobar hemorrhages in conscious patients with hematomas up to 100 ml. Of the 601 total patients, 307 were randomized to early surgical evacuation and were compared to initial standard medical care of 294 patients (of note, if the treating team believed hematoma evacuation was necessary, it was performed at that time). The authors found that 174 of 297 (59%) of the surgical group had an unfavorable outcome compared to 178 of 286 (62%) of the initial medical care group (OR 0.86; 95% CI 0.62–1.2; $P = 0.367$). STICH II was unable to demonstrate a statistical benefit to early hematoma evacuation in lobar hemorrhage.[14]

Neurosurgical open craniotomy was the approach utilized in both STICH I and II. The minimally invasive catheter evacuation (MISTIE III) trial evaluated a minimally invasive approach to the evacuation of large hematomas (>30 ml) to a target of <15 ml. This international, multicenter open-label trial randomized 506 patients to surgical intervention or medical care. A total of 499 patients (250 in the surgical group and 249 in the medical group) were included in the analyses. The authors reported that 45% of the surgical group compared to 41% of the medical group had mRS values of 0–3 at 365 days (adjusted risk difference 4%; 95% CI –4 to 12;

$P = 0.3$). While this minimally invasive approach did improve ICP and cerebral perfusion pressure (CPP) parameters and may have demonstrated a modest mortality benefit (upon secondary subgroup analysis), it did not improve long-term outcomes.[15]

Neurosurgical hematoma evacuation through an open craniotomy or an image-guided minimally invasive catheter approach is not recommended as standard of care at this time. This is an active area of ongoing research.

It is important to appreciate that cerebellar hemorrhages are typically considered for neurosurgical intervention if there is evidence and/or risk of damaging the brainstem.[1,5]

7.9 Differential Diagnoses

The differential diagnosis upon initial presentation is broad. With a good history, brief clinical exam and initial imaging ICH can be elucidated quickly. The underlying etiologies of the ICH include aneurysmal subarachnoid hemorrhage, dural arteriovenous fistulas, venous malformation rupture, hypertension, cerebral amyloid angiopathy, venous sinus thrombosis, neoplasms, intracranial arterial dissection, hemorrhagic transformation of ischemic stroke, and trauma. These can all be complicated by coagulopathy.[1,2,5]

7.10 Complications

ICH is a highly morbid disease and presents both diagnostic and therapeutic challenges. However, once the diagnosis is made, supporting the patient is a multidisciplinary task as numerous complications can change the clinical course. For this reason, frequent neuro checks (clinical neuromonitoring) and neuroimaging (radiographic monitoring) are important and can affect treatment considerations and outcomes.[4]

7.11 Intraventricular Hemorrhage

Intraventricular hemorrhage (IVH) complicates >40% of patients with ICH and is known to increase mortality substantially. Commonly, IVH is associated with locations closely approximated to the ventricular space such as the thalamus. Blood within the ventricular system can lead to hydrocephalus, fever, elevated ICP, and depressed levels of consciousness. These patients often benefit from EVD placement and close monitoring of ICP and CPP variables.[1,2,5]

A double-blind, placebo-controlled, multisite trial (CLEAR IVH III) randomized 500 patients with ICH who had IVH and an indwelling EVD. The study compared 246 patients who received intraventricular alteplase to 245 patients who received intraventricular saline. The authors reported no difference in functional outcome between the two groups (risk ratio 1.06; 95% CI 0.88–1.28; P = 0.55). The group that received alteplase did demonstrate a decrease in mortality but the patients that lived primarily achieved a mRS of 5 (severely devastating disability).[16] Intraventricular hemorrhage is a dangerous complication of ICH; however, routine or protocolized administration of alteplase is not recommended at this time. Future studies are ongoing to address questions of patient selection, dosing, and optimal timing.

7.12 Cerebral Edema and Intracranial Hypertension

Cerebral edema is common in ICH and the amount of edema is closely associated with hematoma size. Hyperosmolar therapy utilizing mannitol, hypertonic saline, or both is the mainstay of pharmacologic intervention to address cerebral edema. There are no specific evidence-based protocols for the initiation, titration, or discontinuation of hyperosmolar therapy for cerebral edema. It is important to note that mannitol use above a serum osmolality of 320 mOsm/kg may increase the risk of renal failure and should be avoided.[5]

Elevations in ICP (>22 mmHg) have been associated with poor outcomes. The detection of ICP can be accomplished with various invasive monitoring such as an EVD, intraparenchymal monitor or subdural monitor. There are a variety of noninvasive techniques that represent areas of active research.[2]

The treatment of the ICP elevation varies according to the underlying cause and appropriate interpretation of the ICP waveforms. The NCS recommends targeting ICP <22 mmHg and maintaining a minimal CPP of 60 mmHg. The CPP is equal to the mean arterial pressure (MAP) minus the ICP. It may be possible to individualize these values for a particular patient based on patient factors such as cerebral oxygen tension.[1,2]

7.13 Neuropsychiatric Complications

Delirium is common and has been shown to negatively impact outcomes in patients with ICH even in the absence of comorbid infection, invasive mechanical ventilation, or medications that are typically associated with delirium. Additionally, the subtype of agitated delirium may confer additional risk of poor outcomes.[17,18] There is no specific guideline-based treatment of delirium in ICH at this time.

Depression has been demonstrated in approximately 20% of patients with ICH. Depression has also been shown to worsen outcomes and is not optimally assessed at all centers. One study that used diagnostic codes as a surrogate for detection of depressive symptoms noted only a minority of ICH patients clearly received treatment for their depressive symptoms. Treatment of underlying depressive symptoms in ICH may represent a unique therapeutic opportunity in a disease that has seen little improvement in outcomes.[19]

7.14 Seizures

The frequency of seizures in ICH is variable in the literature but rates >30% have been reported. Comatose patients are likely at greatest risk. Non-convulsive seizures may represent up to 20% of seizures in ICH patients with impaired consciousness. Continuous electroencephalography (cEEG) is recommended for patients with ICH and impaired consciousness. Documented seizures should be treated and the choice of pharmacologic agent is highly dependent on patient factors and the clinical scenario.[1,2,5]

There are currently no recommendations for the use of prophylactic antiseizure pharmacotherapy. There has been data demonstrating worse outcomes with phenytoin prophylaxis.[2]

7.15 Outcomes

It is important to consider what therapeutic interventions address morbidity and mortality. The mRS is the most commonly utilized outcome tool in ICH studies. It addresses functional status (independence versus dependence) but does not capture quality of life metrics. Other tools such as NeuroQoL, which is a validated set of quality of life questions for patients with neurologic disease, may provide additional insight. The Patient-Reported Outcomes Measurement System has additional tools that address questions that important to patients and caregivers. Yet another tool, the NIH Toolbox, evaluates several domains including cognitive, motor, and emotional health.[5] With these (and other similar) tools, it is easier to take a patient-centered approach to our therapeutic interventions and our communication of prognostication information.

7.16 Conclusion

ICH accounts for less than one-fourth of all strokes, but disproportionately accounts for stroke morbidity and mortality. After ensuring the patient is safe (evaluating ABCs), a careful history and clinical exam can provide the necessary information to pursue appropriate neuroimaging to determine diagnosis and potential etiology of ICH. An initial stat CT scan can differentiate between ischemic and hemorrhagic stroke. The main principles of management of ICH involve addressing hemodynamic abnormalities, reversing coagulopathy, determining severity of illness, and monitoring for and treating complications such as ICP elevations, IVH, seizures, and neuropsychiatric issues. Our conversations about diagnosis and prognosis with patients and families should reflect our respect for outcomes that matter most to patients. This would include mortality but also should include quality of life.

References

1. Claude Hemphill J, Greenberg SM, Anderson CS. AHA/ASA guidelines for the management of spontaneous intracerebral hemorrhage. Stroke. Epub May 22, 2015;46:1–30.
2. Lam AM, Singh V, O'Meara AMI. Emergency neurological life support: intracerebral hemorrhage. Neurocrit Care. Springer US; Epub August 27, 2019;32:1–15.
3. Steiner T, Al-Shahi Salman R, Beer R, Wagner M. European Stroke Organisation (ESO) guidelines for the management of spontaneous intracerebral hemorrhage. Int J Stroke. 2014;9:840–55.
4. Maas MB, Rosenberg NF, Kosteva AR. Surveillance neuroimaging and neurologic examinations affect care for intracerebral hemorrhage. J Neurol. 2013;81:107–12.
5. Naidech AM. Diagnosis and management of spontaneous intracerebral hemorrhage. Continuum (Minneap Minn). 2015;21:1228–98.
6. Kothari RU, Brott T, Broderick JP, et al. The ABCs of measuring intracerebral hemorrhage volumes. Stroke. Lippincott Williams & Wilkins; 1996;27:1304–05.

7. Wada R, Aviv RI, Fox AJ, et al. CT angiography "spot sign" predicts hematoma expansion in acute intracerebral hemorrhage. Stroke. Lippincott Williams & Wilkins; 2007;38:1257–62.

8. Anderson CS, Heeley E, Huang Y, et al. Rapid blood-pressure lowering in patients with acute intracerebral hemorrhage. N Engl J Med. 2013;368:2355–65.

9. Qureshi AI, Palesch YY, Foster LD, et al. Blood pressure-attained analysis of ATACH 2 trial. Stroke. 2018;49:1412–18.

10. Qureshi AI, Palesch YY, Barsan WG, et al. Intensive blood-pressure lowering in patients with acute cerebral hemorrhage. N Engl J Med. 2016;375:1033–43.

11. Baharoglu I, Cordonnier C, Al-Shahi Salman R, et al. Platelet transfusion versus standard care after acute stroke due to spontaneous cerebral haemorrhage associated with antiplatelet therapy (PATCH): a randomised, open-label, phase 3 trial. The Lancet. Elsevier Ltd; 2016;387:2605–13.

12. Naidech AM, Maas MB, Levasseur-Franklin KE, et al. Desmopressin improves platelet activity in acute intracerebral hemorrhage. Stroke. Epub July 8, 2014;45(8):2451–53.

13. Mendelow AD, Gregson BA, Fernandes HM, et al. Early surgery versus initial conservative treatment in patients with spontaneous supratentorial intracerebral haematomas in the International Surgical Trial in Intracerebral Haemorrhage (STICH): a randomised trial. The Lancet. 2005;365:387–97.

14. Mendelow DA, Gregson BA, Rowan EN, et al. Early surgery versus initial conservative treatment in patients with spontaneous supratentorial lobar intracerebral haematomas (STICH II): a randomised trial. The Lancet. Mendelow et al. Open Access article distributed under the terms of CC BY-NC-ND; 2013;382:397–408.

15. Hanley DF, Thompson RE, Rosenblum M, et al. Efficacy and safety of minimally invasive surgery with thrombolysis in intracerebral haemorrhage evacuation (MISTIE III): a randomised, controlled, open-label, blinded endpoint phase 3 trial. The Lancet. Elsevier Ltd; 2019;393:1021–32.

16. Hanley DF, Lane K, McBee N, et al. Thrombolytic removal of intraventricular haemorrhage in treatment of severe stroke: results of the randomised, multicentre, multiregion, placebo-controlled CLEAR III trial. The Lancet. Elsevier Ltd; 2017;389:603–11.

17. Naidech AM, Beaumont JL, Berman M, et al. Dichotomous "good outcome" indicates mobility more than cognitive or social quality of life. Crit Care Med. 2015;43:1654–59.

18. Rosenthal LJ, Francis BA, Beaumont JL, et al. Agitation, delirium, and cognitive outcomes in intracerebral hemorrhage. Psychosomatics. Elsevier; 2017;58:19–27.

19. Francis BA, Beaumont J, Maas MB, et al. Depressive symptom prevalence after intracerebral hemorrhage: a multi-center study. J Patient Rep. Epub November 21, 2018;2:1–7.

8

Correction of Coagulopathy

Ahmed M Salem and Tiffany R Chang

Abstract

Coagulopathy is the loss of balance between hemostatic and fibrinolytic processes resulting in excessive bleeding, intravascular thrombosis, or abnormalities in coagulation testing. It is frequently encountered in the neurocritical care unit and can contribute to poor outcomes. Coagulopathies present unique challenges to the neurointensivist, where early recognition and appropriate management are key. In this chapter, we will discuss techniques to assess coagulopathies as well as treatment strategies for the brain-injured patient.

8.1 Introduction

Coagulopathy may be defined as the loss of balance between hemostatic and fibrinolytic processes, which may result in either excessive bleeding or intravascular thrombosis. Abnormalities in coagulation testing may also be considered evidence of coagulopathy, even in the absence of clinical sequelae of bleeding or thrombosis.

There are limited data on the incidence of coagulopathy in neurocritical care units; however, it is commonly seen in critically ill patients with incidences ranging widely from 14% to 81%. Coagulopathies may be acquired through the use of medications, trauma, and organ failure. Its presence may confer an increased risk of poor functional outcome, hematoma expansion, and death. An aging patient population and increased use of antithrombotic and anticoagulant agents demand unique considerations. Timely, appropriate assessment and treatment are warranted to mitigate hematoma expansion and to facilitate emergent neurosurgical intervention when indicated. In this chapter, techniques in the assessment and management of coagulopathies for the patient with an intracranial hemorrhage will be discussed, in line with the most recent guidelines adopted by the American Heart Association (AHA), American Stroke Association (ASA), Neurocritical Care Society (NCS), and Society of Critical Care Medicine (SCCM),[1,2] as well as updates from recent clinical trial findings.

8.2 Coagulation Assessment

8.2.1 CONVENTIONAL COAGULATION TESTS

Conventional (or common) coagulation tests (CCT) include prothrombin time/international normalized ratio (PT/INR), activated partial thromboplastin time (aPTT), platelet count, D-dimer, and fibrinogen levels. The PT is a laboratory test developed to assess the function of the "extrinsic pathway" whereby calcium and tissue factor (TF) are added to citrated blood plasma and the time to coagulation is measured. To correct for interlaboratory differences in TF preparations, the INR was developed, and was only intended for monitoring the effect of warfarin therapy. Abnormalities in PT may reflect coagulopathy seen in liver failure, disseminated intravascular coagulopathy (DIC), trauma as well as in the case of some medications such as factor Xa inhibitors. The aPTT is commonly used to assess the "intrinsic pathway" of hemostasis and is performed by adding calcium, phospholipid, and an activator such as kaolin to citrated blood plasma, and the time to coagulation is measured. It is most useful for monitoring the effect of unfractionated heparin (UFH); however, it cannot reliably reflect the effect of other anticoagulants.

CCTs present limitations as they are plasma-based and hence cannot measure interactions between clotting factors, TF, and platelets, and were not designed to assess hemostatic integrity in the trauma or preoperative patient; they simply reflect a static evaluation of the coagulation cascade with clot formation as their endpoint rather than assessing the whole coagulation system. They have also been shown to correlate poorly with clinical bleeding and transfusion requirements, lack accuracy in detecting deficiencies in coagulation factors, fail to detect the effects of novel anticoagulation agents or antiplatelet therapy, and do not describe platelet function and fibrinolysis.

8.2.2 VISCOELASTIC HEMOSTATIC ASSAYS

Shortcomings of CCTs have led to increased utilization of viscoelastic hemostatic assays (VHAs), which offer a better depiction of the successive steps that comprise the cell-based theory of hemostasis, that is, initiation, amplification, propagation, and termination through fibrinolysis. VHAs are performed by placing whole blood in a cup with a suspended pin, which transduces changes in tension during clot formation and breakdown with rotation (Figure 8.1a and 8.1b).

Thrombelastography (TEG) is a VHA commonly used in North America. It measures different phases of the coagulation cascade including time to initiate clot formation (reaction time, R), rate of clot formation (kinetics, K; angle, α), maximum clot strength (maximum amplitude, MA), and clot stability (fibrinolysis, Ly30). When compared with CCT, TEG has been shown to be a better predictor of significant bleeding, the need for massive transfusions as well as mortality at 24 h and 30 days following trauma.[3] Furthermore, there is a reported mortality benefit to TEG-directed hemostatic resuscitation in trauma patients requiring massive transfusions when compared to interventions dictated by CCTs.[4,5] Figure 8.2 illustrates suggested CCT and VHA thresholds for blood product transfusions in patients with serious or life-threatening hemorrhage and the corresponding hemostatic agents to use.

(a)

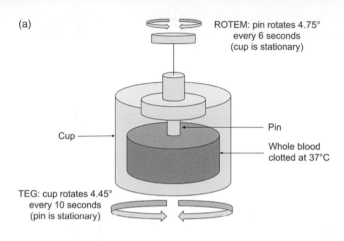

ROTEM: pin rotates 4.75°
every 6 seconds
(cup is stationary)

Cup

Pin

Whole blood
clotted at 37°C

TEG: cup rotates 4.45°
every 10 seconds
(pin is stationary)

(b)

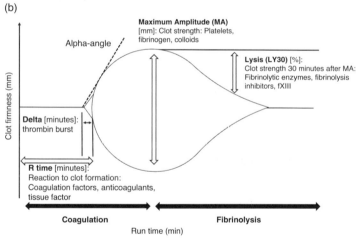

Figure 8.1 (a) Schematic of viscoelastic testing with specimen of whole blood in a cup
warmed to 37°C. With TEG, the cup oscillates with pin remaining stationary, while with
ROTEM pin oscillates while the cup remains stationary. Measurement of pin synchronization
with the cup reflects the stages of clot formation. (b) Thrombelastography recording with
measurement parameters.
Reproduced from review article by Salem et al.[14]

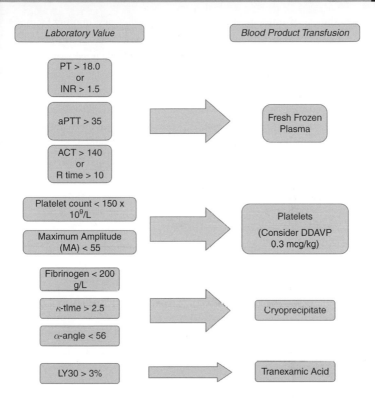

Figure 8.2 Conventional coagulation testing and thromboelastography thresholds are shown along with corresponding hemostatic agents for reversal of coagulopathy in patients with serious or life-threatening hemorrhage.
PT = prothrombin time, aPTT = activated partial thromboplastin time, ACT = activated clotting time, R time = reaction time, Ly30 = percentage lysis at 30 min.

8.2.3 PLATELET FUNCTION

While CCT identifies patients at increased risk of bleeding due to thrombocytopenia, it does not indicate qualitative platelet dysfunction due to the use of antiplatelet therapy, renal insufficiency, or other factors. Bleeding time has grown out of favor for this purpose due to its operator-dependence and lack of sensitivity. The gold standard for assessment of platelet function is considered to be light transmission aggregometry in platelet-rich plasma or whole blood, but availability may be limited due to poor standardization and time consumption. Commercially available point-of-care platelet function assays overcome some of these obstacles and include the platelet function analyzer (PFA-100; Siemens Medical Solutions, Malvern, PA) and VerifyNow (Accumetrics, San Diego, CA) ASA and P2Y12 assays. These tests detect dysfunction secondary to the use of antiplatelets and can provide measures of patient response to these agents as well as adequacy of efforts to reverse them. Standard TEG testing unreliably detects the presence of single antiplatelet therapy (APT) use; however, it may detect coagulopathy seen in combination APT use. TEG with platelet mapping (TEG-PM) (Haemoscope Corporation, Niles, IL) is a specific VHA that has been shown to correlate with platelet aggregometry and is able to detect platelet dysfunction due to APT and other coagulopathies. In neurocritically ill patients, such as those with SAH, ICH, or TBI, platelet dysfunction may be seen even in the absence of APT use or failure of other organ systems and may confer worse outcomes.

8.2.4   FIBRINOLYSIS

Hyperfibrinolysis, while only seen in 2–6% of patients, may have a powerful impact on outcome from major trauma. It has long been recognized as a contributor to the coagulopathy seen in shock and in trauma. While elevations in D-dimer and FDP on CCT may indicate the presence of hyperfibrinolysis, TEG is the only single test that provides information on the balance between thrombosis and fibrinolysis. Ly30 values greater than 3% have been shown to predict the need for massive transfusion and are associated with a 2-fold increase in mortality in trauma patients. It has also been shown that higher degrees of fibrinolysis correlate with all shock parameters and hemorrhage-related mortality.

Coagulopathy following TBI is associated with the severity of injury. In one report, it was present in up to one-third of patients with isolated TBI and up to 60% of patients with severe TBI, although there have been reports of lower rates. The brain is rich in TF and it is postulated that the release of TF activates the extrinsic pathway, which in turn leads to consumptive coagulopathy and hyperfibrinolysis. Hyperfibrinolysis may play an important role in predicting poor outcomes in patients with TBI, with D-dimer at admission shown to be an independent risk factor for poor outcome.

The CRASH-2 and MATTERs trials, which demonstrated a statistically significant mortality benefit in trauma patients with uncontrolled hemorrhage who were treated with antifibrinolytic therapy early in the course of their treatment, have served to highlight the importance of hyperfibrinolysis as a target for therapy. While the subsequent CRASH-3 trial failed to demonstrate a statistically significant difference in the primary outcome of head injury-related death overall, there was a mortality reduction in the subgroup of patients with mild-to-moderate TBI.

The use of antifibrinolytics in spontaneous ICH was examined in the TICH-2 trial, which, despite a statistically significant decrease in the rate of hematoma expansion in the TXA group, failed to demonstrate a difference in functional outcomes.

8.3 Reversal of Antithrombotic Therapy

There has been a significant, continued increase in the use of antithrombotic agents among patients admitted to the neurocritical care unit, due to an aging population and increased diagnosis of ischemic events that warrant such therapies. The introduction of novel agents poses a diagnostic and therapeutic dilemma for the neurointensivist when managing the patient with intracranial hemorrhage. Antithrombotic agents may be roughly divided into antiplatelet therapy (APT) and anticoagulant therapy.

8.3.1 ANTIPLATELET THERAPY

The main classes of antiplatelet drugs commonly used in practice include cyclooxygenase-1 (COX-1) inhibitors (e.g. acetylsalicylic acid, ASA or aspirin), phosphodiesterase (PDE) inhibitors (e.g. dipyridamole and cilostazol), P2Y12 receptor inhibitors (e.g. clopidogrel, prasugrel, and ticagrelor), and glycoprotein IIb/IIIa inhibitors (e.g. abciximab, epitifibatide, and tirofiban).

Single APT use is associated with a low risk of major bleeding, although this risk increases significantly when combination APTs are implemented, similar to the risk of anticoagulants. In a study of a large cohort of patients from the Get With The Guidelines-Stroke (GWTG-Stroke) database with ICH, the use of combination APT, but not single APT, was associated with a higher risk for in-hospital mortality when compared with patients not taking APT.[6]

Reversal of APT in the bleeding patient may be achieved through the administration of platelet transfusion. Routine platelet transfusion for ICH based on reported use of APT alone was associated with an increased rate of poor functional outcome in the PATCH trial.[7] It is important to note that this trial did not utilize qualitative platelet function testing and excluded surgical patients, so platelet transfusion may be appropriate for patients who require neurosurgical intervention. In a study by Choi et al. of 107 patients presenting with traumatic intracranial hemorrhage and reported APT use, a significant percentage of patients had subtherapeutic ASA/P2Y12 assays that would be unlikely to benefit from platelet transfusion. Among patients who did receive platelet transfusions, the amount transfused did not adequately reverse its effect in almost half of this patient cohort.[8] There may, therefore, be a role for targeted platelet transfusions based on quantitative assessment of platelet function before and after transfusion. This was illustrated in a retrospective study by Naidech et al. on a series of patients with ICH and abnormal platelet function activity. Early (<12 h from symptom onset) platelet transfusion improved platelet activity assay results and was associated with smaller final hemorrhage size and more independence at 3 months (modified Rankin score < 4).[9] Similarly, in a TBI population, TEG-directed platelet transfusion was associated with decreased mortality compared to a historical cohort in a retrospective study by Furay et al.[10]

Desmopressin (DDAVP) use has also been demonstrated to improve platelet function in patients on COX-1 and ADP receptor inhibitors in several tests of platelet function compared to those who had not received reversal agents. Clinically, it has been shown to reduce blood loss and improve hemostasis in patients with aspirin exposure undergoing cardiac surgery. In patients with intracranial hemorrhage and either reduced platelet activity on PFA-100 and/or known aspirin use, DDAVP administration has been shown to be associated with restoration of platelet function on repeat testing. Given its low cost and relatively good safety profile, its administration should be considered in patients with intracranial hemorrhage who were exposed to antiplatelet agents.[2]

8.3.2 ANTICOAGULATION THERAPY

The main classes of anticoagulant drugs include vitamin K–dependent coagulation factor antagonists (VKA, e.g. warfarin), factor Xa inhibitors (e.g. fondaparinux, rivaroxaban, apixaban), direct thrombin inhibitors (DTI, e.g. argatroban, bivaluridin, dabigatran), and heparinoids (i.e. unfractionated, or UFH, and low-molecular-weight heparin, or LMWH). In the neurocritical care unit, common indications for these medications include stroke prevention in atrial fibrillation and treatment of venous thromboembolism. Reversal strategies for anticoagulation-associated intracranial hemorrhage are summarized in Figure 8.3.[2]

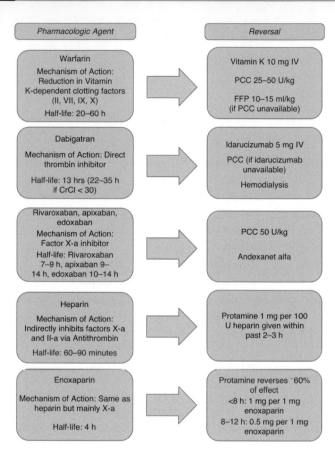

Pharmacologic Agent	Reversal
Warfarin Mechanism of Action: Reduction in Vitamin K-dependent clotting factors (II, VII, IX, X) Half-life: 20–60 h	Vitamin K 10 mg IV PCC 25–50 U/kg FFP 10–15 ml/kg (if PCC unavailable)
Dabigatran Mechanism of Action: Direct thrombin inhibitor Half-life: 13 hrs (22–35 h if CrCl < 30)	Idarucizumab 5 mg IV PCC (if idarucizumab unavailable) Hemodialysis
Rivaroxaban, apixaban, edoxaban Mechanism of Action: Factor X-a inhibitor Half-life: Rivaroxaban 7–9 h, apixaban 9–14 h, edoxaban 10–14 h	PCC 50 U/kg Andexanet alfa
Heparin Mechanism of Action: Indirectly inhibits factors X-a and II-a via Antithrombin Half-life: 60–90 minutes	Protamine 1 mg per 100 U heparin given within past 2–3 h
Enoxaparin Mechanism of Action: Same as heparin but mainly X-a Half-life: 4 h	Protamine reverses ~60% of effect <8 h: 1 mg per 1 mg enoxaparin 8–12 h: 0.5 mg per 1 mg enoxaparin

Figure 8.3 Anticoagulant agents, mechanism, and duration of action along with their corresponding reversal agents

8.3.2.1   Vitamin K Antagonists

VKA inhibit vitamin K–dependent factors in the coagulation cascade: factors II, VII, IX, and X. VKA activity can be assessed by PT/INR. The risk of bleeding while taking a VKA increases with the duration of therapy and higher INR levels. For each increment in INR elevation above the therapeutic range, the risk of bleeding on a VKA doubles.

Vitamin K replacement is essential to replenish the vitamin K–dependent factors and reverse VKA activity. It should be given promptly and IV administration mitigates variability in oral vitamin K absorption. Although the risk profile is low, it may take 24 h or more to become effective.

Fresh frozen plasma (FFP) has been conventionally used to reverse VKA in conjunction with vitamin K. Although it is relatively inexpensive and widely available, its use is complicated by delays in administration, potential transfusion-related reactions, and large volumes that may be required for full INR reversal. This had led to the more widespread use of prothrombin complex concentrate (PCC). PCC is derived from plasma and contains factors II, VII, IX, and X in variable proportions in different preparations. It is rapidly administered in a small volume. PCC has been demonstrated to reverse INR to <1.4 and maintain INR reversal for >48 h in the majority of patients on VKA therapy. In the INCH trial, a randomized trial comparing FFP and PCC for VKA reversal in intracranial hemorrhage, PCC provided more rapid INR reversal with an effective reduction in hematoma expansion.[11] The trial was stopped early due to safety concerns with FFP therapy. Both the AHA/ASA as well as the NCS/SCCM guidelines currently recommend consideration of PCC over FFP for VKA reversal in ICH.[1,2]

8.3.2.2   Factor Xa Inhibitors

Xa inhibitors prevent the conversion of prothrombin to thrombin. Detection of novel agents using calibrated chromogenic assays is expensive and not readily available, and the utility of existing anti-Xa assays have not been validated to identify the presence of the oral factor Xa inhibitors. There are data to support the use of TEG to detect coagulopathies induced by these agents, which may inform reversal strategies in these patients.[12]

PCC is commonly used for Xa inhibitor reversal. PCC has been demonstrated to effectively reverse rivaroxaban in healthy volunteers. In the setting of intracranial bleeding, it is recommended to administer 50 units/kg if the medication was ingested within 3–5 half-lives or if the time of last exposure is unknown. In patients with a known ingestion within 2 h, activated charcoal may also be utilized if this is deemed safe from an airway protection standpoint. Hemodialysis is not effective in removing Xa inhibitors.[2]

Andexanet alfa is a recombinant inactive form of factor Xa. It binds to Xa inhibitors with high affinity and sequesters the medication, resulting in reduced anti-Xa activity. In the ANNEXA-4 study of 352 patients with major bleeding, andexanet alfa reduced anti-Xa levels by 92% in rivaroxaban/apixaban-treated patients and 75% in enoxaparin. Andexanet alfa is approved by the FDA for the reversal of rivaroxaban and apixaban, but widespread use is limited due to the cost of the medication.

8.3.2.3 Direct Thrombin Inhibitors

DTI directly inhibit the activity of factor IIa, which is the key factor in converting fibrinogen to fibrin. DTI have an additional unique indication in the treatment of heparin-induced thrombocytopenia. Intravenous formulations are short acting and generally do not require reversal agents. However, the reversal of oral dabigatran was challenging before idarucizumab became available. Idarucizumab is a monoclonal antibody, which binds to dabigatran with considerably higher affinity than factor IIa. In the RE-VERSE AD study of 503 patients with life-threatening bleeding (Group A) or need for emergent surgical procedure (Group B), idarucizumab reversed thrombin time to normal in 100% of patients and this effect remained relatively stable 24 h after treatment. Normal intraoperative hemostasis was achieved in 92% of the patients in Group B. The rate of thrombotic events in this study was similar to those reported after major surgical procedures or hospitalization for uncontrolled bleeding, and may be attributable to the low rate of reinitiation of anticoagulation. Idarucizumab is administered in two doses of 2.5 g given within 15 min. Activated charcoal is an additional option for dabigatran, similar to Xa inhibitors, and is recommended for consideration in the AHA/ASA as well as the NCS/SCCM guidelines.[1,2]

If idarucizumab is not available, hemodialysis and PCC are alternative options. Dabigatran is renally excreted and is effectively removed by hemodialysis. However, there is a theoretical risk of worsening cerebral edema in patients with mass lesions. The recommended dosing for PCC is 50 units/kg, the same as for Xa inhibitors. Administration of PCC beyond 3–5 half-lives of dabigatran exposure may be considered in patients with renal insufficiency.[2]

8.3.2.4 Heparin and Low-Molecular-Weight Heparin

UFH activates antithrombin III activity, which inhibits factors IIa and Xa. Heparin activity can be assessed utilizing aPTT or point-of-care activated clotting time (ACT). Heparin activity may also be assessed with TEG; shortening of R time with heparinase implicates the presence of heparin in the sample as the cause of coagulopathy. Its effects may be reversed with protamine, which is a naturally occurring protein that binds to heparin and its dosing is outlined in Figure 8.3.

LMWH has a similar mechanism of action but is longer acting and thought to have more predictable pharmacology in the setting of normal renal function. Assessment of LMWH activity requires the use of an anti-FXa assay. Protamine may be used to reverse LMWH activity, but this reversal is incomplete and estimated to be around 60%.[2] A novel approach to LMWH is andexanet alfa. Although this is a potential therapeutic intervention with a possibility of more complete LMWH reversal than with protamine, it is currently not approved for this indication and is still undergoing further study.

8.4 Coagulopathy in Systemic Disease

8.4.1 ACUTE LIVER FAILURE

Acute liver failure is associated with a deficiency of both procoagulant and anticoagulant proteins. While CCT may show an elevated PT/INR in this patient population, studies utilizing TEG and Thrombin Generation assays have demonstrated that these patients may have a normal ability to form clots and may even be hypercoagulable. Using a combination of these tests may provide a better overall assessment of their coagulopathy.

8.4.2 THROMBOCYTOPENIA

Thrombocytopenia may be seen in a variety of conditions encountered in the neurocritical care unit, including sepsis (which is the most common cause of thrombocytopenia in critically ill patients), hypersplenism, disseminated intravascular coagulopathy, blood loss, mechanical fragmentation, medications, bone marrow suppression, and immune-mediated disorders. In a case series by Chan et al. of patients with thrombocytopenia undergoing neurosurgical procedures, a platelet count <100,000/μl was associated with a significant increase in the rate of postoperative hematoma formation when compared with patients with a platelet count >100,000/μl.[13] Current guidelines recommend a transfusion threshold of <100,000/μl for patients with intracranial bleeding or those undergoing a neurosurgical procedure.

8.4.3 DISSEMINATED INTRAVASCULAR COAGULOPATHY

DIC is associated with multiple disease entities encountered in critically ill patients, most commonly due to sepsis, although trauma and malignancy are also common causes encountered in the neurocritical care unit. It is characterized by widespread microvascular thrombosis due to TF expression, leading to massive fibrin deposition, consumption of platelets and coagulation factors, hyperfibrinolysis, hemorrhage, and organ failure. The management of DIC is that of the underlying condition. CCT-guided transfusion may be used if a patient is actively bleeding or is at high risk of intracranial bleeding.

8.4.4 UREMIA

Uremia is associated with an increased risk of hemorrhage secondary to platelet dysfunction. A rising prevalence of chronic kidney disease and the use of renal replacement therapy have led to this being encountered with increasing frequency in the neurocritical care unit as a cause of, or contributing to, intracranial bleeding. DDAVP is the agent most commonly used in the treatment of uremic bleeding and has been shown to reduce bleeding time and normalize hemostasis in patients with uremic platelets undergoing surgery. Its actions are mediated by an increase in endothelial release of von Willebrand factor and platelet membrane glycoprotein expression, which in turn promotes platelet adhesion to the endothelium. It has been shown to restore platelet function within 30 min of administration, though its effects are short-lived at around 3 h. DDAVP dosed at 0.3–0.4 mcg/kg is administered intravenously for this indication and is well tolerated with few reported side effects.

8.5 Conclusions

Coagulopathy is commonly encountered in the neurocritical care unit and poses a challenge to the clinician when managing the patient with intracranial hemorrhage. Utilization of viscoelastic testing has shown great promise in this arena, allowing one to risk stratify patients and guide transfusion requirements. As the widespread use of antithrombotic therapy continues to increase, further development of specific testing for individual medications and targeted reversal agents would improve the management of hemorrhagic complications.

References

1. Hemphill JC 3rd, Greenberg SM, Anderson CS, Becker K, Bendok BR, Cushman M, et al. Guidelines for the management of spontaneous intracerebral hemorrhage: a guideline for healthcare professionals from the American Heart Association/American Stroke Association. Stroke. July 2015;46(7):2032–60.

2. Frontera JA, Lewin JJ 3rd, Rabinstein AA, Aisiku IP, Alexandrov AW, Cook AM, et al. Guideline for reversal of antithrombotics in intracranial hemorrhage: a statement for healthcare professionals from the Neurocritical Care Society and Society of Critical Care Medicine. Neurocrit Care. February 2016;24(1):6–46.

3. Holcomb JB, Minei KM, Scerbo ML, Radwan ZA, Wade CE, Kozar RA, et al. Admission rapid thrombelastography can replace conventional coagulation tests in the emergency department [Internet]. Ann Surg. 2012;256:476–86. Available from: http://dx.doi.org/10.1097/sla.0b013e3182658180

4. Gonzalez E, Moore EE, Moore HB, Chapman MP, Chin TL, Ghasabyan A, et al. Goal-directed hemostatic resuscitation of trauma-induced coagulopathy: a pragmatic randomized clinical trial comparing a viscoelastic assay to conventional coagulation assays. Ann Surg. June 2016;263(6):1051–59.

5. Tapia NM, Chang A, Norman M, Welsh F, Scott B, Wall MJ, et al. TEG-guided resuscitation is superior to standardized MTP resuscitation in massively transfused penetrating trauma patients [Internet]. J Trauma Acute Care Surg. 2013;74:378–86. Available from: http://dx.doi.org/10.1097/ta.0b013e31827e20e0

6. Khan NI, Siddiqui FM, Goldstein JN, Cox M, Xian Y, Matsouaka RA, et al. Association between previous use of antiplatelet therapy and intracerebral hemorrhage outcomes

[Internet]. Stroke. 2017;48:1810–17. Available from: http://dx.doi.org/10.1161/stro keaha.117.016290

7. Baharoglu MI, Irem Baharoglu M, Cordonnier C, Salman RA-S, de Gans K, Koopman MM, et al. Platelet transfusion versus standard care after acute stroke due to spontaneous cerebral haemorrhage associated with antiplatelet therapy (PATCH): a randomised, open-label, phase 3 trial [Internet]. Lancet. 2016;387:2605–13. Available from: http://dx.doi.org/10.1016/s0140-6736(16)30392-0

8. Choi PA, Parry PV, Bauer JS, Zusman BE, Panczykowski DM, Puccio AM, et al. Use of aspirin and P2Y12 response assays in detecting reversal of platelet inhibition with platelet transfusion in patients with traumatic brain injury on antiplatelet therapy. Neurosurgery. January 1, 2017;80(1):98–104.

9. Naidech AM, Liebling SM, Rosenberg NF, Lindholm PF, Bernstein RA, Batjer HH, et al. Early platelet transfusion improves platelet activity and may improve outcomes after intracerebral hemorrhage. Neurocrit Care. February 2012;16(1):82–87.

10. Furay E, Daley M, Teixeira PG, Coopwood TB, Aydelotte JD, Malesa N, et al. Goal-directed platelet transfusions correct platelet dysfunction and may improve survival in patients with severe traumatic brain injury. J Trauma Acute Care Surg. November 2018;85(5):881–87.

11. Steiner T, Poli S, Griebe M, Hüsing J, Hajda J, Freiberger A, et al. Fresh frozen plasma versus prothrombin complex concentrate in patients with intracranial haemorrhage related to vitamin K antagonists (INCH): a randomised trial. Lancet Neurol. May 2016;15(6):566–73.

12. Dias JD, Norem K, Doorneweerd DD, Thurer RL, Popovsky MA, Omert LA. Use of thromboelastography (TEG) for detection of new oral anticoagulants. Arch Pathol Lab Med. May 2015;139(5):665–73.

13. Chan K-H, Mann KS, Chan TK. The significance of thrombocytopenia in the development of postoperative intracranial hematoma [Internet]. J Neurosurg. 1989;71:38–41. Available from: http://dx.doi.org/10.3171/jns.1989.71.1.0038

14. Salem AM, Roh D, Kitagawa RS, Choi HA, Chang TR. Assessment and management of coagulopathy in neurocritical care [Internet]. J Neurocrit Care. 2019;12:9–19. Available from: http://dx.doi.org/10.18700/jnc.190086

Subarachnoid Hemorrhage

H Alex Choi and Swathi Kondapalli

Abstract

This chapter discusses the management of aneurysmal subarachnoid hemorrhage patients. The sections review the epidemiology, risk factors, clinical presentation, grading scales, and important complications.

9.1 Definition

Spontaneous subarachnoid hemorrhage (SAH) is usually caused by rupture of a cerebral aneurysm, leading to hemorrhage into the space between the arachnoid and pia mater, the subarachnoid space.

9.2 Epidemiology

SAH accounts for ~5% of strokes. The global incidence of SAH is estimated at 6.1 per 100,000 persons for 2010, which is down from 10.2 per 100,000 persons since the 1980s.[1]

9.3 Etiology

Etiologies of spontaneous SAH include ruptured intracranial aneurysms, cerebral arteriovenous malformations, vasculitis, reversible cerebral vasoconstriction syndrome, dural venous sinus thrombosis, superficial artery rupture, pituitary apoplexy, sickle cell anemia, infundibulum rupture, and perimesencephalic nonaneurysmal hemorrhage. This chapter predominantly discusses aneurysmal SAH.

9.4 Risk Factors (Table 9.1)

9.5 Clinical Presentation

- Classic presentation is severe/thunderclap headache, "worst headache of life"
- Nausea/vomiting

Table 9.1 Risk factors for aneurysmal subarachnoid hemorrhage[2,3]

Risk factors for aneurysmal SAH
History of previous aSAH
Hypertension
Smoking
Alcohol abuse
Sympathomimetic drugs
Aneurysmal size >7 mm
Female
Age >50 years
African American or Hispanic race
First-degree member with intracranial aneurysm or $\geq$ 2 first-degree relatives affected
Family history of aSAH
Autosomal dominant polycystic kidney disease
Type IV Ehlers–Danlos syndrome

- Meningismus
  - Nuchal rigidity on neck flexion
  - Can have associated positive Kernig or Brudzinski sign
    - Kernig sign: pain in hamstrings on 90° hip and knee flexion followed by knee extension
    - Brudzinski sign: while supine, neck flexion associated with involuntary hip flexion
- New onset seizure
- Cranial neuropathy likely from aneurysmal compression
  - Oculomotor nerve palsy – can present with diplopia from third nerve palsy, eye remains "down and out."
    - Ptosis
    - Dilated nonreactive pupil
  - Optic neuropathy – with nasal quadrantanopia from ophthalmic artery aneurysm compressing on the optic chiasm
  - Facial pain – with cavernous or supraclinoid aneurysms, compression of the ophthalmic or maxillary nerve may present with symptoms mimicking trigeminal neuralgia
- Sudden loss of consciousness and coma
  - Caused by rupture of aneurysm with sudden increase in intracranial pressure, diffuse global ischemia, reduced cerebral blood flow, ictal cerebral infarctions
- Headache leading to progressive alteration in mental status
  - Caused by hemorrhage and progression of hydrocephalus

9.6 Diagnostic Workup

- Lumbar puncture
  - If there is a normal head CT but high clinical suspicion persists, lumbar puncture should be performed to make a diagnosis of SAH.
  - Xanthochromic appearance (can be appreciated on visual inspection) and persistent RBC count (around >100,000 RBCs/mm^3) elevation

between first and fourth tube can aid in diagnosis. CSF protein will be elevated due to blood breakdown products, but glucose can be normal.

- Radiographic studies
  - Noncontrast CT: Within 48 h of SAH onset, it will detect over 95% of cases
    - Blood in the anterior hemispheric fissure can be suggestive of an anterior communicating artery aneurysm
    - Predominant blood in one Sylvian fissure can be associated with a unilateral middle cerebral or posterior communicating artery aneurysm
    - Blood within the prepontine or peduncular cistern can be suggestive of a superior cerebellar or basilar apex aneurysm
  - Noncontrast MRI: Sensitivity for SAH detection on T2FLAIR increases as met-hemoglobin deposition increases, making MRI useful in a subacute setting (> 4 days from onset) as opposed to acute (within 24–48 h).[4]
  - CT angiogram (CTA): In patients with adequate creatinine clearance, CTA can allow for delineation of cerebral arterial anatomy; however, if aneurysm is suspected but not detectable on CTA, digital subtraction angiography is the gold standard.
  - MR angiogram (MRA): Benefit of limiting radiation exposure allows for this modality to be useful as a screening test for patients with ≥ first-degree relatives, prior aSAH, or pregnant patients with suspected SAH. However, it remains dependent on the direction of flow in the aneurysm relative to the magnetic field as well as the size (poor sensitivity for aneurysms < 3 mm diameter).[5]
  - Digital subtraction angiography (DSA): It is the gold standard for detection of aneurysmal subarachnoid hemorrhages. Detects aneurysm in 80–85% of cases; however, if undetectable or evidence of infundibulum, angiography should be repeated to reevaluate intracranial vasculature. DSA allows for identification of aneurysm anatomy to assist with decision-making process of endovascular coiling versus surgical clipping for aneurysm obliteration.

9.7 Classification of Subarachnoid Hemorrhage

9.7.1 CLINICAL GRADING SCALES

The World Federation of Neurosurgical Societies Scale (WFNS) and the Hunt and Hess Grading Scale are based on the clinical presentation of the patient. These scales are important for clinical prognostication of outcomes, commonly used to categorize the clinical severity of the patient quickly. Patients with Grades I, II, and III are considered low-grade patients, and those with Grades IV and V are considered high-grade patients in both scales (Table 9.2).

Table 9.2 Subarachnoid hemorrhage clinical grading scales

Grade	World Federation of Neurosurgical Societies Scale	Hunt and Hess Grade
I	GCS 15 without focal deficit (aphasia and/or motor deficit)	Asymptomatic, or mild headache and slight nuchal rigidity
II	GCS 13–14 without focal deficit	Moderate to severe headache, nuchal rigidity, cranial nerve palsy only
III	GCS 13–14 with focal deficit	Drowsiness, confusion, or mild focal deficit
IV	GCS 7–12 with or without focal deficit	Stupor, moderate to severe hemiparesis Possible early decerebrate rigidity and vegetative disturbances
V	GCS 3–6 with or without focal deficit	Deep coma, decerebrate rigidity, moribund appearance

9.7.2 RADIOGRAPHIC GRADING SCALES

Radiographic grading scales are used to categorize the amount of subarachnoid blood on a CT brain. The amount of blood is associated with the risk of vasospasm. Fisher Grade 3 carries the highest risk for vasospasm. (Table 9.3) A modified Fisher Scale of 4 carries the highest risk for vasospasm. (Table 9.4)

9.8 Initial Management

As in any medical emergency, the initial focus should be on basic life support, including the ABCs. Often the basics have been performed

Table 9.3 Fisher scale for SAH

Grade	CT Findings
1	No detectable subarachnoid hemorrhage
2	Diffuse SAH, no localized clot > 3 mm thick, OR vertical layers > 1 mm thick
3	Localized clot > 5 × 3 mm in subarachnoid space OR vertical thickness > 1 mm
4	Intraparenchymal or intraventricular hemorrhage with either absent or minimal SAH

Table 9.4 Modified Fisher scale for SAH

Grade	CT Findings
1	Thin SAH with no IVH
2	Thin SAH with bilateral IVH
3	Thick SAH with no IVH
4	Thick SAH with bilateral IVH

Table 9.5 Subarachnoid hemorrhage early brain edema score (SEBES) (Figure 9.1)[6]

Grading scale between 0 and 4
- One point each assigned for
  o absence of visible sulci caused by effacement of sulci or
  o absence of visible sulci with disruption of gray-white matter
- Visualize each hemisphere at two levels on CTH to assess and determine points:
  o Level of insular cortex showing thalamus and basal ganglion above basal cistern
  o Level of centrum semiovale above the level of the lateral ventricle
    For each point increase there were 2.24 times increase in the odds of developing DCI (delayed cerebral ischemia) and 3.2–3.4 times increase in the odds of an unfavorable outcome.

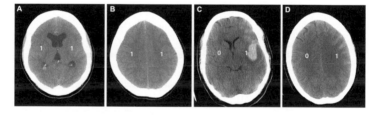

Figure 9.1 SEBES grading (Table 9.5): Grade 4 of SEBES with the effacement of sulci at two predetermined levels in each hemisphere (A and B), and grade 2 of SEBES with the effacement sulci on the left hemisphere (C and D)

prior to the diagnosis of SAH, as this usually requires a CT scan after the initial assessment. In high-grade patients, the airway has been secured. The BP should be supported with vasopressors if necessary, to maintain perfusion.

The initial management of SAH

(1) Mitigate risk of rebleeding
(2) Treat hydrocephalus
(3) Seizure prophylaxis

9.8.1 REBLEEDING

Re-rupture of an aneurysm is associated with poor neurologic outcomes. Initial management to decrease this risk is vital.

- Risk of rebleeding is highest in the first 2–12 h with occurrence rate anywhere from 4% to 13.6% in the first 24 h.[2]
- Factors associated with rebleeding:
  - Persistent systolic blood pressures over 160 mmHg
  - Worsening neurological status
  - Previous sentinel headaches lasting over 1 hr
  - Larger size of aneurysm
  - Extended time to aneurysm treatment

Management should be initiated immediately after diagnosis.

- Goal is to decrease systolic blood pressure under 160 mmHg. Titratable intravenous medications are recommended.
  - Nicardipine
    - Dihydropyridine calcium channel blocker
    - Start at rate of 5 mg/h IV and titrate up by 2.5 mg/h every 5–15 min to achieve SBP goal
    - Maximum dose of 15 mg/h
  - Labetalol
    - Nonselective β-receptor antagonist with post-synaptic α-1-receptor antagonist
    - 10–20 mg IV Push, to be administered over 1–2 min
    - May be repeated once but afterwards should consider starting a titratable infusion

- Infusion usually starts at 1 or 2 mg/min and titrated to desired blood pressure
- Maximum total dose 300 mg, usual total dose 50 mg to 200 mg
  ○ Clevidipine
    - 1–2 mg/h IV 1–2 mg/h IV, titratable every 2–5 min by doubling dose to achieve desired blood pressure
    - Maximum dose of 21 mg/h
- Anti-fibrinolytic medications may be helpful in decreasing risk of re-bleeding. Patients with no medical contraindications can be administered Tranexamic acid, 1-gram bolus with 1 gram every 8 h as an infusion until aneurysm is secured. Aminocaproic acid, which is a competitive inhibitor of plasminogen and plasmin, has also been used to reduce early rebleeding risk. Administration dose is usually 4–5 grams bolus followed by 1 g/h with a maximum of 30 grams per day.
- If anti-fibrinolytic medications are to be used, they should be started as soon as possible as the risk of re-rupture is highest early on and should be limited to 72 h or until aneurysm treatment. The risk of thrombotic events is increased in those treated with anti-fibrinolytic medications.

9.8.2   HYDROCEPHALUS

Obstructive hydrocephalus occurs because of intraventricular hemorrhage and nonobstructive hydrocephalus occurs because of blockage of CSF re-absorption mechanisms. In patients with decreased consciousness (lower GCS scores), agitation, or confusion, an EVD should be considered.

- Acute symptomatic hydrocephalus should be managed by placement of an external ventricular drain (EVD).
- An EVD should be placed in high-grade patients for hydrocephalus management and monitoring of intracranial pressures (ICP).

- After EVD placement, drain should be open at a level of 20 mmHg to decrease the theoretical risk of abruptly decreasing intraventricular pressure, increasing risk of re-rupture of aneurysm.

9.8.3   SEIZURE PROPHYLAXIS

The risk of seizures after SAH is unclear with reported incidence of about 2% after invasive treatment with higher incidence post-clipping versus post-coiling.[7] However, treatment with prophylactic antiepileptics is controversial. The incidence of seizures at ictus is especially difficult to estimate as patients are not being observed and posturing movements from a sudden increase in ICP can be interpreted as seizures by a bystander witness. Treatment with antiepileptic medications is appropriate, especially before the aneurysm is secured. Long-term antiepileptic medication use is not recommended unless patient develops seizures during the disease course.

- Risk factors for the development of early seizures in SAH include history of hypertension, aneurysm in the middle cerebral artery, thickness of SAH clot, associated intracerebral hematoma, rebleeding, and history of stroke.
- Early seizure prophylaxis is recommended for SAH to prevent secondary injury or rebleeding from an unsecured aneurysm.[7] Antiepileptic medications commonly used include Levetiracetam 500 mg twice a day or Dilantin 300 mg daily.
- Long-term use of antiepileptic medications is not recommended unless patient has a seizure.

9.8.4   NEUROGENIC STUNNED MYOCARDIUM

Cardiovascular support is an important clinical consideration in high-grade SAH patients. During the initial event of aneurysmal rupture, a subsequent catecholamine surge leads to hypercontraction of cardiac myocytes, subendocardial ischemia, and as a result, impaired cardiac function. In acute cardiogenic shock, patient will experience hypotension and flash pulmonary edema. Troponins elevations are common.[8]

- Initial management of cardiogenic shock may involve vasopressor support with norepinephrine drip; avoid pure alpha agonists like phenylephrine.
- Intubation and mechanical ventilation may be necessary for oxygenation in the cases of severe flash pulmonary edema.
- Heart function usually resolves within the first days and need for cardiogenic shock usually improves. Ejection fraction improves usually in the first couple of weeks.
- EKG findings can include QT prolongation, high R-wave, deep symmetric T-wave inversion, and peaked P-waves.
- Transthoracic echocardiogram in these states demonstrates intact basal function, moderate-to-severe dysfunction mid ventricle, and apical akinesis or dyskinesis with significantly decreased left ventricular ejection fraction. This imaging finding of the left ventricle has been given the name "Takatsubo cardiomyopathy", referring to the takatsubo fishing pot used in japan to trap octopus.[9]

9.9 In-Hospital Management

All aneurysmal SAH patients should be admitted to the intensive care unit, ideally to a dedicated neurointensive care unit with neurointensivists and neurosurgeons with expertise in SAH care. The mainstays of hospital management include early aneurysm treatment, monitoring for secondary neurologic deterioration, and treatment of those complications.

9.10 Aneurysm Treatment

Early aneurysm treatment is the most effective method of preventing rerupture.[10] It is recommended that the aneurysm is secured within 24–

36 h of admission to the hospital. The method to secure the aneurysm is a patient and practitioner specific decision. Surgical aneurysm clipping may be favored for locations that are more amenable to a surgical approach, for example, middle cerebral artery with extensive subarachnoid hemorrhage. Most institutions have favored endovascular approaches.

- ISAT (international subarachnoid hemorrhage aneurysm trial)
  - Results showed an absolute risk reduction of poor outcomes at 1 year for coiling (23.7%) compared to clipping (31%, p = 0.0019); however, rebleeding rates for coiling were higher than clipping though not statistically significant.
  - Criticisms of the trial include limited randomization, inclusion of mostly low-grade SAH patients (80% were Hunt and Hess grades 1 and 2), and 97% of aneurysms in anterior circulation.[11,12]

9.11 Endovascular versus Surgical Clipping

- Surgical clipping
  - Favorable factors:
    - High neck-to-dome ratio (wide-neck aneurysm)
    - Large (>15 mm) or giant (>24 mm) aneurysm
    - Anterior circulation aneurysms
    - SAH associated with intraparenchymal hemorrhage needing evacuation
    - Symptoms due to mass effect may have better resolution
- Endovascular coiling
  - Favorable for posterior circulation aneurysms
  - Carries lower mortality than clipping

9.12 Complications

9.12.1 DELAYED CEREBRAL ISCHEMIA (DCI) AND CEREBRAL VASOSPASM

- Diagnosis of DCI is usually associated with arterial vasospasm and clinical features of focal neurological signs such as aphasia, hemiparesis, or decreased level of consciousness.[13] However, it can be clinically diagnosed even without angiographic evidence of vasospasm.
- Thirty percent of aSAH patients develop vasospasm, of which up to 20% proceed to have secondary ischemic strokes.
- Arterial vasospasm can occur anywhere from Day 4 to Day 14 post-aSAH. Thirty percent of all patients develop SAH. Oral nimodipine has been shown to improve 90-day functional outcomes, but not reduce risk of vasospasm.
- Prophylactic balloon angioplasty or hypervolemia prior to development of vasospasm is not associated with reduced morbidity.[14]

9.12.2 MONITORING FOR VASOSPASM

Methods of monitoring for the occurrence of vasospasm and risk for DCI vary depending on institution and patient situation.

- Transcranial Dopplers
  - Allows for a noninvasive method of identifying and following vasospasm. Measurements of velocities are used to determine areas of increased flow velocity that is related to narrowed vessel diameter. Pitfalls include availability as well as operator dependent variability in ultrasound utilization.
  - For MCA velocities, mild spasm is defined as >120 cm/s, moderate >160 cm/s, and severe >200 cm/s.

- Lindegaard ratio (LR) is defined as the mean velocity in MCA divided by mean velocity in ipsilateral extracranial ICA. This ratio is usually under three; however, it is used to distinguish whether the MCA velocity is secondary to hyperemia (can also result in flow velocities > 120 cm/s) or vasospasm.
  - LR < 3, suggestive of hyperemia, 3–6 mild vasospasm, > 6 severe vasospasm.
  - By utilizing noninvasive TCD monitoring institutions can provide alternative means of monitoring for signs of early vasospasm.
- CT angiography/CT perfusion
  - Though evidence has been supportive of diagnostic accuracy of CT angiography as a screening test for vasospasm, high contrast injection variability, and inability to detect distal arterial spasm limits its use. CT perfusion has been used to predict patients at high risk for DCI; however, clear thresholds have not been established, and use is limited.
- Cerebral angiography
  - Remains the gold standard test to detect vasospasm; however, the use of cerebral angiography must be considered against its risks, including but not limited to vascular injury, secondary embolic infarctions, contrast, and radiation exposure. In most cases, DSA allows for diagnostic and immediate therapeutic interventions for cerebral vasospasm.
- Continuous EEG monitoring
  - Although limited in availability, continuous quantitative EEG monitoring is used to identify the ratio of alpha to delta waves to detect changes in cerebral blood flow suggesting early detection of vasospasm mediated cerebral ischemia.

9.12.3 STRATEGIES TO PREVENT DCI

- Start oral nimodipine on Day 0 for all aSAH patients.
  - Usually administered as 60 mg q4 h or 30 mg q2 h while maintaining a CPP of 60–70.

- Trials of several agents have been attempted, including magnesium, statins, and clazosentan, which have all failed to reduce DCI rates.
- Maintain euvolemia and avoid fever.

9.12.4   TREATMENT OF DCI

In the setting of suspected DCI, hemodynamic augmentation should begin immediately, while simultaneously ruling out other causes of neurologic deterioration (hydrocephalus, infection, seizures, etc.). Maintain euvolemia and augment blood pressure through fluid resuscitation. Consider starting vasopressors to induce arterial hypertension, which increases cerebral perfusion. Administer vasopressors (norepinephrine is preferred, but phenylephrine and vasopressin can be used as well) to increase SBP by increments of 15% until neurologic improvement is achieved. Complications of hemodynamic augmentation can include exacerbating or causing pulmonary edema and myocardial infarction.

- Elevation of SBP by increments of 15% until SBP 220 or side effects of hypertension are seen.
- Cerebral angiography with balloon angioplasty or intra-arterial vasodilation with administration of intra-arterial nicardipine/verapamil/milrinone/nitroglycerin either as a single agent or in combination can be used. Intra-ventricular nicardipine can be used to induce intraventricular vasodilation.
- Intravenous milrinone can be used for refractory cases. Care should be taken to avoid hypotension.
- Complications of hemodynamic augmentation can include exacerbating or causing pulmonary edema, hemorrhagic transformation of a previous ischemic area, and myocardial infarction.

9.12.5   HYDROCEPHALUS MANAGEMENT

EVD placement and CSF diversion is an important part of initial management. The appropriate management and timing of EVD weaning is more controversial.[15] EVDs can be kept at a specific level usually 20 mmHg or 10 mmHg and allowed to drain freely, or EVDs can be kept clamped with intermittent drainage for elevated pressures. No clear consensus exists. Additionally, the appropriate time and method of weaning an EVD is controversial. Some advocate for an aggressive strategy, rapid weaning over 1–2 days and others, slow prolonged weaning over several days.

- EVD weaning should be considered once patient is stable neurologically, generally after concerns for vasospasm and increased ICP have passed.
- To mitigate the risk of EVD infection, EVDs should be weaned as soon as possible.
- EVD weaning can occur rapidly within 1–2 days.
- Chronic symptomatic hydrocephalus should be treated with permanent flow diversion, via ventriculoperitoneal, ventriculoatrial, or lumboperitoneal shunt.

9.12.6   HYPONATREMIA FOLLOWING SAH

Hyponatremia (serum sodium level <135 mEq/L) is commonly seen in SAH. The cause is associated with altered plasma and CSF concentration of natriuretic peptide causing the cerebral salt wasting. The phenomenon is associated with hyponatremia and auto-diuresis. Clinical volume status, which is at times difficult to assess, is the differentiating factor between cerebral salt wasting and the syndrome of inappropriate antidiuretic hormone. Patients with cerebral salt wasting are clinically hypovolemic and patients with SIADH are clinically euvolemic. In general, the treatment for hyponatremia after SAH is to replete sodium levels with hypertonic

solutions. Fluid restriction after SAH to treat SIADH should be performed
with extreme caution as to avoid hypovolemia, which can precipitate DCI.

- Goals for management remain maintaining normonatremia (135–
  145 mmol/L) and euvolemia.
- Administration of IV fluids either as hypertonic (2% or 3%) or as
  isotonic solutions with additional salt tablets can be used to manage
  hyponatremia and volume status.[16]

9.12.7   FEVER

Central fever has been associated with volume of hemorrhage, severity of
injury, and development of vasospasm. Although fever after SAH has been
associated with poor outcomes, it is unclear if aggressive fever control is
associated with improved outcomes. The general recommendation is to
avoid fever with conventional methods of acetaminophen, cooling blanket
as tolerated. Aggressive fever control with invasive cooling catheters or
external cooling gel pads is performed but not proven to improve outcomes.

- Conservative measures; that is, acetaminophen and cooling blankets
  are recommended.
- Aggressive measure with external gel pad or catheter-based cooling
  technology can be used with caution.

9.12.8   ANEMIA

In patients at risk for cerebral ischemia or DCI, red blood cell transfusions
in anemic patients have been associated with improved outcomes after
SAH.[17]

- No consensus has been identified on ideal hematocrit goals;
  however, some have advocated for a hemoglobin value above 10 in
  those with symptoms of DCI or vasospasm.[2]
- Recently more liberal transfusion thresholds are used such as
  above 8 or 9.

9.12.9 PROGNOSIS AND RECURRENCE RATES

Incidental aneurysms without aSAH have expected bleeding rates based on size and location. Aneurysms under 7 mm in diameter have an annual bleed risk of 0.1% per year, and greater than 12 mm about 3% bleed rate per year. Between 7 and 12 mm, anterior circulation aneurysms have a bleed rate of about 0.5% per year, and posterior circulation aneurysms about 3% per year.

Aneurysms that are incompletely treated either by endovascular coiling or by surgical clipping are always at risk of increasing in size or rebleeding. The risk of recurrence of a clipped aneurysm that is completely treated is about 1.5% at 4 years.[18]

Improved treatment modalities, early aneurysm treatment, and the development of neurocritical care units have improved overall survival of rates after SAH.[19] However, we are increasingly becoming aware of long term cognitive dysfunction, psychological disease and sexual dysfunction as important symptoms, which can be disabling and lead to poor quality of life along with increase in familial and economic burden. Most prevalent in cognitive disability includes memory dysfunction and psychomotor recovery, though all aspects of cognitive dysfunction can persist.[19,20]

References

1. Etminan N, Chang HS, Hackenberg K, et al. Worldwide incidence of aneurysmal subarachnoid hemorrhage according to region, time period, blood pressure, and smoking prevalance in the population (a systematic review and meta-analysis). JAMA Neurol. 2019;76(5):588–97.
2. Connolly ES Jr., Rabinstein AA, Carhuapoma JR, et al. American Heart Association Stroke Council, Council on Cardiovascular Radiology, Intervention, Council on Cardiovascular Nursing, Council on Cardiovascular Surgery, Anesthesia, Council on Clinical Cardiology. Guidelines for the management of aneurysmal subarachnoid hemorrhage: a guideline for healthcare professionals from the American Heart Association/American Stroke Association. Stroke. 2012;43:1711–37.

3. Eden SV, Heisler M, Green C, Morgenstern LB. Racial and ethnic disparities in the treatment of cerebrovascular diseases: importance to the practicing neurosurgeon. Neurocrit Care. 2008;9:55–73.

4. van der Kleij LA, De Vis JB, Olivot JM, et al. Magnetic resonance imaging and cerebral ischemia after aneurysmal subarachnoid hemorrhage: a systemic review and meta-analysis. Stroke. 2017;48:239–45.

5. White PM, Wardlaw JM, Easton V. Can noninvasive imaging accurately depict intracranial aneurysms? A systematic review. Radiology. 2000;217:361–70.

6. Ahn SH, Savarraj JP, Pervez M, et al. The subarachnoid hemorrhage early brain edema score predicts delayed cerebral ischemia and clinical outcomes. Neurosurgery. 2018;83:137–45.

7. Lanzino G, D'Urso PI, Suarez J, et al. Seizures and anticonvulsants after aneurysmal subarachnoid hemorrhage. Neurocrit Care. 2011;15:247.

8. Naidech AM, Kreiter KT, Janjua N, et al. Cardiac troponin elevation, cardiovascular morbidity, and outcome after subarachnoid hemorrhage. Circulation. 2005;112 (18):2851–56.

9. Wittstein IS, Thiemann DR, Lima JAC, et al. Neurohumoral features of myocardial stunning due to sudden emotional stress. N Engl J Med. 2005;352:539–48.

10. Lantigua H, Ortega-Gutierrez S, Schmidt JM, et al. Subarachnoid hemorrhage: who dies, and why? Crit Care. August 31, 2015;19(1):309.

11. Molyneux AJ, Kerr RS, Yu LM, et al. International subarachnoid aneurysm trial (ISAT) of neurosurgical clipping versus endovascular coiling in 2143 patients with ruptured intracranial aneurysms: a randomised comparison of effects on survival, dependency, seizures, rebleeding, subgroups, and aneurysm occlusion. Lancet. 2005;366 (9488).809–17.

12. Bederson JB, Awad IA, Wiebers DO, et al. Recommendations for the management of patients with unruptured intracranial aneurysms: a statement for healthcare professionals from the Stroke Council of the American Heart Association. Circulation. 2000;102:2300–08.

13. Vergouwen MD, Vermeulen M, van Gijn J, et al. Definition of delayed cerebral ischemia after aneurysmal subarachnoid hemorrhage as an outcome event in clinical trials and observational studies: proposal of a multidisciplinary research group. Stroke. 2010;41:2391–95.

14. Zwienenberg-Lee M, Harman J, Rudisill N, et al., Balloon Prophylaxis for Aneurysmal Vasospasm (BPAV) Study Group. Effect of prophylactic transluminal balloon angioplasty on cerebral vasospasm and outcome in patients with Fisher grade III subarachnoid hemorrhage: results of a phase II multicenter, randomized, clinical trial. Stroke. 2008;39:1759–65.

15. Klopfenstein JD, Kim LJ, I. Feiz-Erfan I, et al. Comparison of rapid and gradual weaning from external ventricular drainage in patients with aneurysmal subarachnoid hemorrhage: a prospective randomized trial. J Neurosurg. 2004;100:225–29.

16. Al-Rawi PG, Tseng MY, Richards HK, et al. Hypertonic saline in patients with poor-grade subarachnoid hemorrhage improves cerebral blood flow, brain tissue oxygen, and pH. Stroke. 2010;41:122–28.

17. Naidech AM, Drescher J, Ault ML, et al. Higher hemoglobin is associated with less cerebral infarction, poor outcome, and death after subarachnoid hemorrhage. Neurosurgery. 2006;59(4):775–80.

18. Naidech AM, Janjua N, Kreiter KT, et al. Predictors and impact of aneurysm rebleeding after subarachnoid hemorrhage. Arch Neurol. 2005;62:410–16.

19. Lovelock CE, Rinkel G, Rothwell P, et al. Time trends in outcome of subarachnoid hemorrhage: population-based study and systematic review. Neurology. 2010;74 (19):1494–501.

20. Mayer SA, Kreiter KT, Copeland D. Global and domain-specific cognitive impairment and outcome after subarachnoid hemorrhage. Neurology. 2002;59(11):1750–58.

10

Subdural Hematoma

Peter Pruitt

Abstract

Subdural hematoma (SDH) is the most common form of traumatic intracranial hemorrhage. SDH occurs in the potential space between the dura and arachnoid membranes. Initial presentation ranges from asymptomatic to coma, with subacute and chronic SDH often having more insidious presentations. Diagnosis is most commonly via non-contrast head CT scan. Treatment includes surgical drainage, reversal of anticoagulation, and supportive care.

10.1 Background and Epidemiology

Subdural hematoma (SDH) is defined as bleeding that occurs between the dura and arachnoid membranes, outside of the brain parenchyma. It is distinguished from epidural hematomas (EDH), the other major type of extra-axial hematoma, which are formed between the dura and the skull. Major risk factors for SDH include older age and use of anticoagulants and antiplatelet agents.[1]

Timing of SDH plays an important role in prognostication and management of SDH. From the onset of symptoms, SDH can be divided into:

- Acute SDH: 0–2 days from onset or traumatic injury.
- Subacute SDH: 3–14 days after onset or traumatic injury.
- Chronic SDH: 15+ days from onset or traumatic injury.

10.2 Pathophysiology

There are multiple potential etiologies for SDH. Most SDH occur due to the disruption of the bridging veins that connect the dural sinuses to the surface of the brain, secondary to trauma. Additionally, SDH can also occur in the setting of arterial rupture; these may represent between 30 and 50% of SDH.[2] In post-procedural patients (e.g. lumbar puncture or surgery), intracranial hypotension can cause increased pressure on the bridging veins, causing them to burst and leading to SDH. Other rarer causes include aneurysmal rupture (including aneurysmal SAH).

In patients with cerebral atrophy (e.g. elderly patients, patients with a history of alcohol abuse), the space between the dura and the brain tissue becomes wider, increasing tension on the bridging veins and causing them to rupture after even minor trauma. Therefore, in these patients, the history of trauma may not be readily apparent. Acute SDH in younger patients is associated with more severe traumatic brain injuries and may portend a poorer prognosis.

After the initial disruption of the bridging veins (or less commonly arteries), bleeding continues until a clot forms, or enough pressure builds up that the wound tamponades. If enough blood extravasates into a fixed space, it will put pressure on the surrounding brain tissue. Shifting of the brain leads to depressed mental status and coma due to increased intracranial pressure (ICP), potentially causing decreased cerebral perfusion pressure.

Some SDHs will resorb without intervention, some will form subdural hygromas, whereas some will liquefy and then enlarge, becoming chronic SDH. Subdural hygromas form over two weeks: first, a capsule is noted to form around the hematoma, and then there is increased vascularity. Some chronic SDH will have recurrent acute bleeding, known as acute-on-chronic SDH.

10.3 Presentation

The presentation of SDH can be widely varied, depending on the severity and chronicity of the injury. Up to 50% of patients with acute SDH will present with coma.[3] Patients with acute posterior fossa SDH may present with vomiting, cranial nerve deficits, cerebellar symptoms, and headache referable to the location of the SDH. Smaller acute SDHs may present asymptomatically after head trauma, or with headache, confusion and other symptoms suggestive of concussion.

The presentations of patients with chronic SDH are more varied and may simply present with headache or global cognitive dysfunction. Patients can also have focal neurologic deficits (e.g. hemiparesis, speech deficits) if there is compression – most commonly contralateral from direct compression but can also be ipsilateral secondary to midline shift.

10.4 Evaluation

10.4.1 INITIAL IMAGING

For the initial imaging of patients with suspected SDH, non-contrast head CT scan is the imaging test of choice. MRI can evaluate for dural neoplasms in spontaneous SDH, but otherwise has a limited role in the initial evaluation of these patients.[4] Providers can also consider non-invasive angiography (CTA or MRA) in spontaneous SDH without a clear source of bleeding to evaluate for an anatomic source.

10.4.2 REPEAT IMAGING

The utility of routine, repeat head CT imaging in SDH is unproven in non-comatose patients. Repeat CT scan at 6 h is a common practice, while other institutions instead recommend repeat imaging only when dictated by changes in the neurologic examination, such as confusion or coma.

10.4.3 IMAGING INTERPRETATION

When evaluating an extra-axial hematoma, SDH will typically not cross
suture lines (e.g., at the falx) – this makes the SDH appear crescent shaped.
In contrast, EDH will not cross dural attachments, so it will be lentiform.
Hematomas can present in one or both of the cerebral convexities, the falx
or tentorium, or the posterior fossa.

Acute SDH will show up as a high-density fluid collection, reflecting
the density of acute intracranial bleeding. These are usually readily
identifiable (see Figure 10.1). Subacute SDH typically appear isodense to
hypodense (after Day 10) – these can be very difficult to identify, especially
if there are bilateral collections.[5] Chronic SDH should appear hypodense,
sometimes with septations, and will have a similar intensity to CSF.

10.4.4 OTHER PROCEDURES

As with any space-occupying intracranial lesion, lumbar puncture is
generally contraindicated because the resulting decrease in infratentorial
pressure may lead to an increase in the volume of SDH.

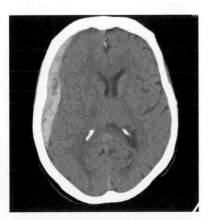

Figure 10.1 Acute parafalcine
subdural hematoma

10.5 Clinical Management

10.5.1 INTRACRANIAL PRESSURE MONITORING

ICP elevation is associated with both increased mortality and worsened functional outcome in patients with SDH. Because of this, management of elevated ICP is crucial, especially for patients who will undergo subsequent surgical drainage.

The most important clinical signs of elevated intracranial pressure are those associated with brainstem herniation, including depressed level of consciousness, extensor posturing, and pupillary abnormalities (e.g. dilation). These are signs that should be addressed with pharmacologic and surgical interventions to reduce ICP (described later).

Based on level II evidence, ICP monitoring is recommended for all patients with SDH and depressed consciousness, defined as a Glasgow Coma Scale (GCS) < 8.[3] However, the presence of SDH may obviate the placement of an intracranial pressure monitor, and reductions in ICP from cerebrospinal fluid drainage may inadvertently lead to an increase in SDH volume.

10.5.2 SURGICAL INTERVENTION

Symptomatic acute SDH is typically managed with neurosurgical drainage. Due to the liquefied nature of chronic SDH, these can often be managed with burr hole drainage and insertion of a Jackson–Pratt drain.

For acute SDH, the most common guidelines recommend surgical drainage with hematoma thickness >10 mm or midline shift >5 mm, if the GCS score decreases by ≥2 points after injury, or for patients with asymmetric or fixed and dilated pupils.[3] For patients with preserved consciousness, CT elements predicting need for surgical intervention include increasing hematoma thickness, presence of acute-on-chronic hematoma, and presence of midline shift on CT scan.[6,7]

Early operative management (within 2–4 h) may have reduced mortality when compared with delayed neurosurgery in observational studies, and so earlier operation is recommended.[3]

10.5.3   MEDICAL THERAPIES

10.5.3.1   Anticoagulation Reversal

Most patients diagnosed with SDH who are on anticoagulation should have their anticoagulation stopped and reversed; however, this should be done on a case-by-case basis that considers the original indication for their anticoagulation and the potential consequences of ending this therapy. For all patients, it is important to check laboratory values, including international normalized ratio (INR), prothrombin time (PTT), and assays that identify antithrombic medication (e.g., platelet activity assays, anti-Xa levels), depending on the anticoagulant used. In general, a normal INR (e.g., <1.5) is desirable.

Most patients with symptomatic SDH should have their anticoagulation reversed, but the severity and risk of deterioration of the SDH must be weighed against the indication for anticoagulation and risks of reversal.

Warfarin should be reversed using four-factor prothrombin complex concentrate (PCC) and vitamin K administration, or fresh frozen plasma (FFP) if PCC is not available. FFP has substantial associated volume, so administration should be carefully monitored in patients with a history of heart failure. Coagulopathy with warfarin can be assessed using an INR.

Enoxaparin reversal can be attempted with protamine sulfate, although the effectiveness is somewhat limited. Coagulopathy with Heparin can be reversed with protamine; reversal of low-molecular-weight heparin with protamine should be considered, based upon the dose and time from last dose.

Direct oral anticoagulants have varying reversal agents and half-lives. Direct Xa inhibitors (rivaroxaban and apixaban) should be reversed with andexanet alfa if available, or a four-factor PCC if not. The half-life of apixaban is 8–15 h, while the half-life of rivaroxaban is 5–9 h in healthy individuals, but 11–13 h in the elderly. The presence of direct Xa inhibitors and the degree of coagulopathy can be assessed with an anti-Xa level. Given the high cost of both PCC and andexanet alfa, consider evaluating for coagulopathy on laboratory testing if outside the half-life window, especially in clinically stable patients. Dabigatran should be reversed with idarucizumab, a monoclonal antibody (a PCC is a reasonable substitute if idarucizumab is not available). The half-life of dabigatran is 14–17 h.

10.5.3.2   Treatment of Platelet Dysfunction

Patients currently taking aspirin or P2Y12 inhibitors (e.g. clopidogrel, prasugrel, ticagrelor) are at increased risk of bleeding and SDH expansion. However, platelet transfusions have not been shown to be useful in the treatment of medication-induced platelet dysfunction and may have an increased risk of death in other forms of intracranial hemorrhage. They, therefore, are not recommended in patients with SDH.[8] Although based on limited evidence, a single dose of desmopressin (0.4 µg/kg IV) could be considered for patients on antiplatelet medications, although its pharmacological efficacy is better established for aspirin than P2Y12 inhibitors.[9]

10.5.3.3   Seizure Prophylaxis

Patients with acute SDH and depressed consciousness may have up to a 24% risk of seizure, which is substantially reduced after treatment with seizure medications.[10] Utility of seizure medications in patients with acute SDH and preserved consciousness or chronic SDH is less clear. Therefore, seizure medications are less commonly used in these groups.

Fosphenytoin and levetiracetam have similar efficacy,[11] though the simpler dosing and narrower side-effect profile of levetiracetam have led to the increasing use of levetiracetam instead of fosphenytoin. Seizure prophylaxis should be administered for 7 days (extrapolated from the treatment of patients with neurotrauma), at which point it can be stopped unless a seizure has occurred.

Prophylactic dose levetiracetam is generally administered with a loading dose of 20 mg/kg intravenous (IV) rounded to the nearest 250 mg, followed by a maintenance dose of 0.5 – 1 g every 12 h for 7 days.

Fosphenytoin is generally dosed with a loading dose of 17–20 mg phenytoin equivalents (PE)/kg IV, with a maximum dose of 2 g, followed by a maintenance dose of 5 mg PE/kg/day in divided doses every 8 h for 7 days. Fosphenytoin levels should be carefully monitored in patients with hepatic or renal disease, as clearance may be affected. Fospheyntoin should be administered slowly (no more than 150 mg PE per min) due to the risk of cardiovascular side effects, including severe arrhythmias and hypotension.

In patients with SDH and depressed consciousness, consider obtaining continuous EEG monitoring to exclude the presence of subclinical seizures.

10.5.3.4   Corticosteroids

There is no indication for corticosteroid use in patients with acute subdural hematoma. There have been several retrospective studies about the use of corticosteroids (typically dexamethasone) for the treatment chronic subdural hematoma, and there are ongoing trials studying this issue. Given the absence of evidence, there is no clear consensus about whether treatment with steroids is beneficial at the time of writing.

10.5.3.5   Medical Management of Elevated ICP

In the event of clinical signs of brainstem herniation (e.g., unilateral pupillary dilatation, worsening coma, or extensor posturing), immediate treatment of elevated ICP is required. The most effective strategy for ICP management is immediate surgical decompression, if offered.

However, there are several immediate interventions that can be undertaken prior to surgical intervention, or if intervention is not possible. Elevating the head of bed to 30° is a simple, immediate, bedside intervention. Additionally, it is important to remove items that could be constricting the neck and therefore obstructing venous drainage, such as a cervical collar. For brief periods, there may be some benefit to hyperventilation aiming for a $PaCO_2$ of 30 mmHg.

Hyperosmolar therapy is a useful medical intervention to reduce ICP. There has been no demonstrated benefit to treating to a defined target sodium level or serum osmolarity. Therefore, the following treatment regimen is recommended:

- Hypertonic saline: If the patient appears hypovolemic, treat with 30–120 ml of 23.4% hypertonic saline. This infusion should be administered preferably via central venous access. A bolus of 250 ml of 3% hypertonic saline is a reasonable alternative, and does not typically require central venous access.
- In patients who have volume overload or have heart failure, treat with mannitol between 1.0 and 1.5 mg/kg, tending toward higher doses, which have been shown to have improved outcomes.

Both hypertonic saline and mannitol can be used in combination in critically ill patients with imminent or ongoing herniation. Importantly, pharmacologic therapy generally delays the need for more definitive surgical decompression and may not obviate the need for it.

10.5.3.6 Sedation and Analgesia

Prior meta-analyses have not found any significant evidence favoring one sedative agent over another in patients with severe neurotrauma.[12] For intubated patients, sedation regimens can be chosen based on hospital protocols for brain-injured patients. Potential first-line agents for sedation include propofol or dexmedetomidine, while fentanyl is the most frequent first-line analgesic agent.

10.5.3.7 Ventilatory Support

Ventilatory support in patients with SDH is managed similarly to patients with other forms of traumatic brain injury. The primary goals of ventilatory support in patients include avoidance of hypoxia and hypercapnia. Ensure adequate sedation, typically with propofol or dexmedetomidine, with the goal of sedating toward ventilatory synchrony and hemodynamic stability. Propofol is a particularly attractive agent for patients with SDH due to the short half-life, allowing for rapid neurologic assessment in patients with fluctuating mental status. Hypercapnia is common with the use of low-tidal volume lung-protective ventilation, so these strategies should only be used in patients where the ICP can be monitored to ensure that hypercapnia is not causing increased ICP.

10.5.3.8 Hypothermia

Most evidence shows similar to slightly worse outcomes for SDH patients treated with hypothermia. Hypothermia is currently not recommended for patients with SDH.[9]

10.6 Prognosis

Acute SDH has a relatively high in-hospital mortality – up to 55% in some studies. As expected, patients with lower GCS scores at presentation tend to have worse outcomes. On the other hand, patients with preserved consciousness – GCS 13 to 15 – tend to do well, with mortality of about 1% and surgical intervention rates between 10 and 15%.[6,7] Patients with other concurrent forms of hemorrhage (subarachnoid hemorrhage, contusion) tend to have worse outcomes compared with patients with SDH alone.

10.7 Recurrence

While acute SDH will sometimes progress to chronic SDH, the risk of recurrent acute SDH is very low. Chronic SDH have a higher rate of recurrence, with recurrent hematoma occurring in between 5 and 30% of patients.

References

1. Gaist D, Garcia Rodriguez LA, Hellfritzsch M, Poulsen FR, Halle B, Hallas J, et al. Association of antithrombotic drug use with subdural hematoma risk. JAMA – J Am Med Assoc. 2017;317(8):836–46.

2. Maxeiner H, Wolff M. Pure subdural hematomas: a postmortem analysis of their form and bleeding points. Neurosurgery. 2002;50(3):503–09.

3. Bullock MR, Chesnut R, Ghajar J, Gordon D, Hartl R, Newell DW, et al. Surgical management of acute subdural hematomas [Internet]. Neurosurgery. March 2006;58(Suppl 3): S16–24; discussion Si-iv. Available from: www.ncbi.nlm.nih.gov/pubmed/16710968

4. Carroll JJ, Lavine SD, Meyers PM. Imaging of subdural hematomas [Internet]. Neurosurg Clin N Am. 2017;28(2):179–203. Available from: http://dx.doi.org/10.1016/j.nec.2016.11.001

5. Scotti G, Terbrugge K, Melancon D, Belanger G. Evaluation of the age of subdural hematomas by computerized tomography. J Neurosurg. 1977;47(3):311–15.

6. Pruitt P, Ornam J Van, Borczuk P. A decision instrument to identify isolated traumatic subdural hematomas at low risk of neurologic deterioration, surgical intervention, or radiographic worsening [Internet]. Acad Emerg Med. November 2017;24(11):1377–86. Available from: http://www.ncbi.nlm.nih.gov/pubmed/28871614

7. Orlando A, Levy AS, Rubin BA, Tanner A, Carrick MM, Lieser M, et al. Isolated subdural hematomas in mild traumatic brain injury. Part 1: the association between radiographic characteristics and neurosurgical intervention [Internet]. J Neurosurg. 2018;130(5):1–10. Available from: https://thejns.org/doi/abs/10.3171/2018.1.JNS171884

8. Nishijima DK, Zehtabchi S, Berrong J, Legome E. Utility of platelet transfusion in adult patients with traumatic intracranial hemorrhage and preinjury antiplatelet use [Internet]. J Trauma Acute Care Surg. June 2012 [cited December 5, 2016];72 (6):1658–63. Available from: www.ncbi.nlm.nih.gov/pubmed/22695437

9. Al-Mufti F, Mayer SA. Neurocritical care of acute subdural hemorrhage [Internet]. Neurosurg Clin N Am. 2017;28(2):267–78. Available from: http://dx.doi.org/10.1016/j.nec.2016.11.009

10. Temkin N, Dimken S, Wilensky A, Keihm J, Chabal S, Winn R. A randomized, double-blind study of phenytoin for the prevention of post-traumatic seizures. N Engl J Med. 1990;323(8):497–502.

11. Radic JAE, Chou SH-Y, Du R, Lee JW. Levetiracetam versus phenytoin: a comparison of efficacy of seizure prophylaxis and adverse event risk following acute or subacute subdural hematoma diagnosis [Internet]. Neurocrit Care. October 2014;21(2):228–37. Available from: https://doi.org/10.1007/s12028-013-9951-x

12. Roberts DJ, Hall RI, Kramer AH, Robertson HL, Gallagher CN, Zygun DA. Sedation for critically ill adults with severe traumatic brain injury: a systematic review of randomized controlled trials. Crit Care Med. 2011;39(12):2743–51.

11

Critical Care Management of Neurotrauma

Giang T Quach and Michael Shapiro

Abstract

The critical care management of neurotrauma patients is very complex, requiring a strong knowledge base in both neurology and trauma surgery. This chapter is designed as a bridge for healthcare providers from different specialties, including residents and fellows, hospitalists, ICU physicians, and advanced practice providers seeing patients with neurotrauma in an intensive care unit setting, to be more familiar managing common issues encountered in this patient population. The chapter addresses core knowledge in trauma surgery, such as the ABCDE approach in trauma assessment, cervical spine management, hemorrhagic shock, the reversal of anticoagulants, chest tube management, abdominal and extremity compartment syndrome, and burn. The chapter also offers introductory comments about head injury, management of traumatic brain injury (TBI), intracranial hemorrhage (ICH), and intracranial pressure (ICP).

11.1 Initial Assessment: ABCDE of Trauma[1]

11.1.1 A: AIRWAY

- If the patient can communicate verbally, the airway is likely patent, though if the patient is altered or in shock, it may not be adequate.

- Patients who have a GCS equal to or less than 8 should have an airway established. If there is any doubt regarding the patient's ability to maintain an airway, a definitive airway should be established.
- When assessing and managing the airway, including during intubation, inline immobilization of the cervical spine should be maintained to prevent excessive movement, including hyperflexion, hyperextension, or rotation.
- A cervical collar should be in place in suspected cervical injury, including any blunt injury above the clavicle or blunt multisystem trauma. Removal of a cervical collar should occur, ideally, after both clinical and radiographic assessment.
- If the cervical collar must be removed temporarily, a member of the trauma team should manually stabilize the head and neck using inline immobilization.

11.1.2   B: BREATHING

- The patient's chest and neck should be examined for jugular venous distension, tracheal deviation, or asymmetric chest wall excursion. These findings may be associated with pneumothorax, hemothorax, and flail chest.
- Breath sounds should be equal bilaterally with symmetric chest wall rise.
- If pneumothorax or hemothorax is suspected, immediate intervention with needle decompression or tube thoracostomy must be performed.

11.1.3   C: CIRCULATION WITH HEMORRHAGE CONTROL

- Hypotension in a trauma patient should be considered hemorrhagic shock until proven otherwise. Inability to measure the blood pressure should indicate that the patient is hypotensive, not that there is a mechanical difficulty with the blood pressure cuff.

- Palpate and identify the presence of distal pulses (radial, femoral, or dorsalis pedis).
- Identify sources of life-threatening bleeding. Intervention may include direct pressure or packing of wounds, placement of a tourniquet on an extremity, and placement of a pelvic binder.
- Chest X-ray is useful to identify massive hemothorax. Ultrasound examination (FAST), diagnostic peritoneal lavage (DPL), and computerized tomography (CT) may diagnose torso hemorrhage requiring operation. Unstable patients with torso injury are likely to need an operation for hemorrhage control; prompt evaluation by a surgeon is essential.

11.1.4   D: DISABILITY (NEUROLOGIC EVALUATION)

- Quick neurologic evaluation is performed including assessment of level of consciousness, pupillary size and reaction, lateralizing signs, and spinal cord injury level.
- Glasgow Coma Scale (GCS) should be calculated. The best motor response is the most important component.
- The main goal of initial management is to identify primary brain injury and prevent secondary brain injury by ensuring adequate oxygenation and perfusion.

11.1.5   E: EXPOSURE AND ENVIRONMENTAL CONTROL

- All clothes should be removed for complete examination from head to toes, front and back.
- Hypothermia must be avoided. The patient should be covered with warm blankets, or a warming device should be employed.

11.2 Cervical Spine Management

11.2.1 CERVICAL SPINE COLLAR INDICATION

11.2.1.1 The NEXUS Clinical Criteria

The presence of any one of the following findings is clinical evidence that a patient is at increased risk for cervical spine injury and requires radiographic evaluation(CT scan):

- Tenderness at the posterior midline of the cervical spine
- Focal neurologic deficit
- Decreased level of alertness
- Evidence of intoxication
- Clinically apparent pain that might distract the patient from the pain of a cervical spine injury.

11.2.1.2 Canadian C-Spine Rule

- There are high-risk and low-risk factors as below:
  - High-risk factors:
    - Age 65 or above
    - Numbness/tingling in extremities
    - Dangerous mechanism, including fall from ≥3 ft (0.9 m)/5 stairs, axial load injury (diving), high-speed motor vehicle collision (MVC) or with rollover or ejection, bicycle collision, and motorized recreational vehicle (ATV).
  - Low-risk factors:
    - Sitting position in the ED
    - Ambulatory at any time
    - Delayed (not immediate onset) neck pain, no midline tenderness
    - Simple rear-end motor vehicle collision (MVC) (not simple if pushed into traffic, hit by bus/large truck, rollover, hit by a high-speed vehicle).
- If the patient has one of the high risks, evaluate the C-spine with CT scan.

- If the patient has no high risks and no low risks, evaluate the C-spine with CT scan.
- If the patient has no high risks but meets one of the low-risk factors, it is safe to assess if the patient is able to rotate their neck 45° to left and right even with some pain, then no further imaging is needed.

11.2.2 WHEN TO CLEAR CERVICAL COLLAR[2]

- In awake, alert patients with no neurologic deficit or distracting injury, no neck pain or tenderness with full range of motion, cervical spine (CS) imaging is not necessary and cervical collar may be removed.
- In patients with suspected CS injury, pain or tenderness, neurologic deficit, AMS and distracting injury, CT cervical spine should be obtained.
- If CT demonstrates injury, maintain cervical immobilization and consult the spine surgery team.
- If CT is negative in a neurologically intact, awake and alert patient who is complaining of neck pain, an MRI of the spine is recommended to assess for ligamentous injury (note: the incidence of this is low enough to make the recommendation uncertain, but it reflects the authors' current practice). If all imaging is normal, the spine can be cleared, although a hard or soft collar may be offered for comfort.
- If CT is negative in an obtunded patient but without suspicion for spinal cord injury, MR is recommended to complete the evaluation. If the patient cannot undergo MR then maintenance of the hard collar is recommended until either the patient can be examined clinically (i.e. awake and reliable), or pending reevaluation by CT scan at 4 weeks.

11.2.3 HOW TO "CLEAR" THE CERVICAL SPINE

- Examiner stands at the head of the bed.
- Remove anterior collar while patient maintains neutral head position.

- Palpate posterior cervical midline to assure no tenderness.
- Ask the patient to rotate their head left and right, then extend and flex the neck.
- If there is no pain to palpation and with full active range of motion, the cervical collar may be removed. If the patient has pain on any movement, stop and replace the cervical collar. Additional imaging (MRI) may be needed.

11.3 Hemorrhagic Shock

11.3.1 CLASSIFICATION OF HEMORRHAGIC SHOCK (TABLE 11.1)[3]

Note that hypotension does not reliably occur until Class III (more than 1.5 l of blood loss).

11.3.2 RESUSCITATION WITH CRYSTALLOIDS AND COLLOIDS

- Initial fluid bolus of 1 l of Lactated Ringers or 0.9 normal saline (NS) for adults.

Table 11.1 Classification of hemorrhagic shock

	I	II	III	IV
Blood loss (ml)	<750	750–1,500	1,500–2,000	>2,000
Blood loss (%)	<15	15–30	30–40	>40
Heart rate (bpm)	<100	**Tachycardia (>100)**	>120	>140
Blood pressure	Normal	Normal/Orthostatic	**Hypotension**	Severe hypotension
Mental Status	Normal	Anxious	Confused	Altered

- "Permissive hypotension": balancing the goal of organ perfusion with risk of bleeding, not necessary to achieve normotension. This is primarily intended as a temporizing strategy for patients with hemorrhage who cannot immediately go to surgery for definitive control. It may be inappropriate for patients with head injury.
- Transfusion should be balanced between packed red blood cells (PRBC), fresh frozen plasma (FFP), and platelets, i.e. a 1:1:1 ratio of blood products.
- Consider tranexamic acid (TXA) in bleeding patients: 1 g in 50 ml NS IV over 10 min, then 1 g/250 ml NS over 8 h. TXA is safe in patients with TBI, and treatment within 3 h of injury reduces head injury-related death.[4]
- Assess the patient's response by identifying adequate end-organ perfusion and oxygenation (heart rate, blood pressure, urine output > 0.5 ml/kg, level of consciousness, peripheral perfusion, lactate level, base deficit).
- Response to the initial fluid bolus is indicative of the patient's status:
  - **Rapid Response:** Hemodynamically stable after initial fluid bolus. These patients are unlikely to require emergent operative intervention. Radiographic evaluation of injuries should continue with surgical consultation. Blood should be cross-matched for use if necessary.
  - **Transient Response:** Responds to initial fluid bolus but deteriorates again after completion. These patients should have further resuscitation with blood products and are likely to require surgery (or angio-embolization).
  - **No Response:** These patients require resuscitation with blood products (consider activation of a massive-transfusion protocol), should receive TXA, and are most likely to require immediate intervention to control hemorrhage (surgery or angio-embolization).

11.3.3 REVERSAL OF ANTICOAGULANTS

11.3.3.1 Important Factors to Consider

- Type of anticoagulant
- Time since last dose
- Current labs: CBC, PT (INR)/PTT, fibrinogen, antiXa level, thromboelastography (TEG)
- Urgency of reversal
- Risks vs. benefits of reversal

11.3.3.2 Denovo Anticoagulants (Direct Xa Inhibitor)

Consider 5 half-lives as time for the drug to be eliminated (Tables 11.2 and 11.3).

11.3.3.3 Unfractionated Heparin (UFH)

- Half-life 1–1.5 h.
- Subcutaneous heparin (prophylaxis) does not need reversal.

Table 11.2 Reversal of denovo-anticoagulants (direct Xa Inhibitor)

Drug	Half life (h)	5 half-lives (days)	Clearance	Reversal Agent	Dosing
Dabigatran (Pradaxa)	12–17	2.5–3.5	Renal	Idarucizumab (Praxbind)	5 g
Rivaroxaban (Xarelto)	5–9	1–2	Renal/ hepatic	Andexanet alfa (AndexXa) OR 4-factor	See dosing AndexXa below
Apixaban (Eliquis)	8–15	1.5–3	Renal/ hepatic	Prothrombin Complex Concentrates (Kcentra, Otaplex)	50 units/kg

Table 11.3 Dosing of coagulation factor Xa recombinant (AndexXa)

Drug	Strength of last dose	Time since last dose		Dosing of AndexXa	
		<8 h	≥ 8 h	Low dose	High dose
Rivaroxaban	≤10 mg	Low dose	Low dose	400 mg @	800 mg @
(Xarelto)	>10 mg or unknown	High dose		30 mg/min then 4 mg/	30 mg/min then 8 mg/
Apixaban	≤5 mg	Low dose		min for	min for
(Eliquis)	>5 mg or unknown	High dose		120 min	120 min

Table 11.4 Protamine dosing

Time from last dose	Protamine dose (mg) to reverse 100 units of UFH
Less than 30 min	1
30 min to 2 h	0.5
More than 2 h	0.25

- Protamine to reverse systemic heparin (IV push should not exceed 5 mg/min, as rapid administration can cause hypotension and anaphylaxis).

11.3.3.4   Low-Molecular-Weight Heparin (Enoxaparin)

- Half-life 2–8 h.
- Protamine does not reverse LMWH as effectively as UFH.
- Dose 1 mg per 1 mg if enoxaparin was administered within 8 h.
- If more than 12 h has elapsed since last dose, then no protamine is needed (Table 11.4).

11.3.3.5 Warfarin (Coumadin) (Table 11.5)

Half-life 36 h, 5 days for INR to normalize.

11.3.3.6 Antiplatelet Agents

- 10–12% circulating platelets are replaced every day.
- Desmopressin (DDAVP) is used with impaired platelet function in uremia (Hemodialysis patients) (Table 11.6).

Table 11.5 Warfarin (coumadin) reversal

Agent	On Set	Dosing
Phytonadione (Vitamin K)		5–10 mg
PO	24 h	
IV	12 h	IV is associated with risk of anaphylaxis
FFP (least preferred)	2–6 h	10-30 ml/kg
		1 unit FFP ~ 250 ml, *large volume required*
		Short half-life, may repeat dosing in 6 h
PCC (recommended in urgent reversal, consider addition of Vitamin K)	<30 min	INR 1.7–4: 25 u/kg
		INR 4–6: 35 u/kg
		INR >6 50 u/kg, max. dose 500 units

Table 11.6 Reversal of antiplatelet agents

Antiplatelet agents	Half life	Platelet recovery (days)	Reversal Agent
Aspirin	15–20 min	5–10	DDAVP 0.3 mcg/kg IV
Clopidogrel (Plavix)	8 h	~5	over 15 min
Prasugrel (Effient)	7 h	~7	Platelet transfusion
Ticagrellor (Brillinta)	9 h	~3	

11.4 Chest Tubes

11.4.1   CHEST TUBE DRAINAGE SYSTEM

Contemporary devices incorporate the elements of the three-bottle
system, with three chambers: collection, water seal, and suction control
(Figure 11.1).

11.4.1.1   Suction (A)

• Usually set at –20 mmHg (may be increased up to –40 mmHg if there is
  sustained air leak or unresolved pneumothorax).

• Removal of suction ("water seal") is appropriate when pneumothorax
  and air leak have resolved.

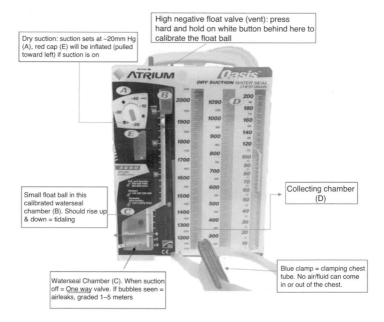

Figure 11.1 Chest tube drainage system (Atrium)

11.4.1.2 Water Seal (C)

This establishes a one-way valve. Air cannot enter the pleural space from the environment but can escape from the pleural space through the chest tube. Air leaving the chest will appear as bubbles in the water seal chamber ("air leak").

11.4.1.3 Collecting Chamber (D)

There are three columns for fluid drainage from the chest.

11.4.2 CHEST TUBE BASICS

11.4.2.1 Waterseal

No suction. This is appropriate when pneumothorax has resolved, even if there is still fluid drainage from the chest.

11.4.2.2 Clamping the Chest Tube

Air and fluid cannot escape the pleural space. If a patient has pneumothorax, a clamped chest tube can lead to tension pneumothorax. This should only be done for a short period of time (may be useful to assess for change in a small residual pneumothorax). If there is any change in the patient's status, the tube should be immediately unclamped.

11.4.2.3 Tidaling

Indicates air movement in the tube with change in thoracic pressure with respiration. The fluid column (and floatball in waterseal column B) should rise and fall with respiration. If tidaling does not occur, the tube may be kinked, clamped, clogged, or displaced outside of the pleural space, and it is unlikely to be functioning.

11.4.2.4 Adjusting Chest Tube

A chest tube can be withdrawn and resecured if it is too far into the chest, but should <u>never</u> be advanced further into the chest. If the tube needs to be advanced it should, instead, be removed and a new tube placed at a new site.

11.4.2.5   Assessing the Chest Tube on Chest X-Ray

Assure that the tube is within the pleural space by confirming that the last hole on the tube, visualized as a break in the radio-opaque line on chest X-ray, is within the thorax. A tube that is directed into a pleural fissure is less likely to remain functional.

11.4.3   Troubleshooting an Air Leak

- Air leaks may be caused by a persistent pneumothorax and by extrinsic breaks in the drainage system. Obtain a chest X-ray to assess the pleural space. Check the insertion site and all tubing connections.
- Clamp the chest tube, briefly.
  - If air leak persists, there is most likely a leak in the collection system. The connection between the chest tube and the collecting system tube is the most common location for an extrinsic leak.
  - If there is no leak in the collection system, then assess the skin entrance site. The wound may require suture or occlusive dressing.

11.4.4   MANAGEMENT OF CHEST TUBE IN TRAUMA

- Chest tube should be placed on suction initially.
- Per ATLS guidelines, consider thoracotomy if initial chest tube output is greater than 1.5 l or more than 200 ml/h during the first 2–4 h after placement.
- Chest tube should be removed as soon as appropriate.
  - Pneumothorax: resolution of pneumothorax and air leak.
  - Hemothorax: output less than ≤ 200 ml/day and thorax clear by chest X-ray.[5]
  - Chest tube may be placed to water seal or clamped prior to removal. If clamped, the patient should be monitored closely for hemodynamic or respiratory difficulty, in which case the tube should be unclamped immediately.

- Chest tube may be removed in ventilated patients. CXR obtained between 1–3 h after removal is sufficient to identify recurrent pneumothorax.

11.5 Abdominal Compartment Syndrome (ACS)

11.5.1 DEFINITION

- ACS is an increase in intraabdominal pressure (abdominal hypertension) that results in a physiologic change via end-organ damage, such as low urine output (renal vein occlusion), hypotension (decreased preload and cardiac output), and hypoxemia/ hypoventilation (increased trans-thoracic pressure).
- Abdominal hypertension is considered when bladder pressure is >12 mmHg, but usually, ACS does not develop until bladder pressure is >25 mmHg. In general, intervention is needed when pressure >35 mmHg.[6,7]

11.5.2 CAUSE

ACS is associated with intraabdominal injury (hemorrhage), reperfusion injury, massive fluid resuscitation and, less commonly, ascites accumulation.

11.5.3 MEASURING ABDOMINAL PRESSURE

Abdominal pressure is usually measured using the urinary bladder pressure as surrogate. Manometry is performed via an indwelling bladder catheter. Measurement is most precise when the patient is intubated and pharmacologically paralyzed, eliminating the confounding effect of abdominal wall tension and muscular contraction. True abdominal compartment syndrome is unlikely in a patient whose respiratory status is not compromised enough to require positive pressure ventilation support.

11.5.4 TREATMENT

The only treatment for true Abdominal Compartment Syndrome is fascial decompression, generally performed through a midline abdominal incision. Abdominal decompression may be performed in the OR or at the bedside in the ICU depending on the patient's level of instability. In those very rare instances where ACS is due to massive free intraperitoneal fluid, it may be possible to achieve decompression by percutaneous drainage.

11.6 Evaluation of Head Injury

11.6.1 CT HEAD INDICATION: CANADIAN CT HEAD RULE (CCTHR)[8]

- Exclusion criteria: Coagulopathy (on anticoagulants or bleeding disorder), <16 years of age, seizure activity
- CT when one of these risks present:
    - GCS <15, 2 h post injury
    - Suspected open or depressed skull fracture
    - Sign of basilar skull fracture (hemotympanum, "racoon" eyes, otorrhea/rhinorrhea, Battle's sign)
    - Vomiting >2 times
    - Age >65 years
    - Amnesia before impact >30 min
    - Dangerous mechanism: Pedestrian struck by motor vehicle, ejected from the vehicle, fall >3 feet/5 stairs

11.6.2　REPEAT CT HEAD

- In minimal head injury (mild TBI), repeat CT head is indicated in the presence of neurologic deterioration or coagulopathy (on anticoagulants or antiplatelet agents).[9–11]
- For moderate or severe TBI, CT head should be repeated within 24 h.

11.6.3　FOCAL INTRACRANIAL INJURY

11.6.3.1　Epidural Hematoma (EDH)

- Usually convex or lenticular in shape.
- Usually involves injury to the middle meningeal artery.
- There may be a "lucid interval" between the time of injury and neurologic deterioration (i.e. don't be overly reassured by a good neurologic exam!).
- Surgical evacuation when EDH >30 ml or for acute EDH and coma (GCS score ≤8) with pupillary abnormalities (anisocoria).

11.6.3.2　Subdural Hematoma (SDH)

- Usually bleeding from bridging veins.
- Shape follows the contour of the brain and crosses the suture lines.
- Can cause midline shift and need for surgical evacuation.

Surgical consideration

- SDH >10 mm in thickness or midline shift >5 mm.
- GCS score is ≤8.
- GCS score has decreased by ≥2 points from the time of injury to hospital admission.
- Asymmetric or fixed and dilated pupils.
- Intracranial pressure (ICP) measurements consistently >20 mmHg.

11.6.3.3 Contusion and Intracerebral Hematoma (Parenchymal Hemorrhage)

- Focal contusions can evolve into coalescent contusion and cause mass effect (brainstem compression), obliteration of the fourth ventricle, effacement of basal cisterns, and obstructive hydrocephalus. Consider the need for surgical evacuation.
- Consider repeat CT scan within 6 h to demonstrate stability of hemorrhage, and consider additional scans depending on clinical course.

11.7 Traumatic Brain Injury (TBI)

11.7.1 DEFINITION

- TBI may be defined as a disruption or alteration of brain structure or function by external mechanical forces.[12]
- Primary injuries occur at the time of the accident, such as contusion and hematoma.
- Secondary injuries are those that occur after the initial impact. These injuries occur due to hypoxemia, ischemia, seizures, fever, and hypoglycemia.
- The goal of neurocritical care is to maximize the patient condition to prevent secondary injuries.

11.7.2 CLASSIFICATION

TBI is classified based on Glasgow Coma Scale score (Table 11.7).

Minor	GCS score 13–15
Moderate	GCS score 9–12
Severe (coma)	GCS score 3–8

Table 11.7 Glasgow Coma Scale

Best eye response	Open spontaneously	4
	Open to voice	3
	Open to pain	2
	None	1
Best verbal response	Oriented	5
	Confused	4
	Discernible words	3
	Incomprehensible words/sounds	2
	None	1
Best motor response	Obey commands for movements	6
	Localize to painful stimulus	5
	Withdraw from pain	4
	Decorticate posturing (abnormal flexion)	3
	Decerebrate posturing (abnormal extension)	2
	None	1

11.7.3 MANAGEMENT OF MINOR BRAIN INJURY (GCS 13–15)

- Most minor TBI recovers uneventfully.
- CT scan should be obtained if patient had loss of consciousness for more than 5 min or retrograde amnesia more than 30 min (Section 11.6.1).

11.7.3.1 Outpatient Observation

- If CT head is negative and patient is asymptomatic, the patient can be observed for 4–6 h, and discharged if there are no neurologic abnormalities.
- Ideally, the patient should be discharged with a family member/friend for 24-h observation at home.
- Instructions should include to return to ED if the patient declines in mental status or develops any neurologic deficit.

11.7.3.2   Inpatient Admission

- Patient remains symptomatic but with GCS <15.
- Abnormal CT head.
- Seizures.
- Coagulopathy.
- Neurologic deficit.
- Recurrent vomiting.
- Worsening headache, focal neurologic signs, confusion, and lethargy are highly suggestive of an evolving intracranial hematoma. Around 6–10% of mild TBIs can be complicated by cortical contusions or development of intracranial hemorrhage (intracerebral, subdural, epidural, or subarachnoid).
- In secondary hemorrhage and deterioration with GCS, TBI should be reclassified as moderate or severe.

11.7.3.3   Neurosurgery Consult

The following findings require neurosurgical consultation:
- Mass effect (basal cistern compression or midline shift), sulcal effacement, or herniation.
- Substantial epidural or subdural hematoma (>1 cm in width, or causing mass effect).
- Substantial cerebral contusion (>1 cm in diameter, or more than one site).
- Extensive subarachnoid hemorrhage, posterior fossa, intraventricular, or bilateral hemorrhage.
- Depressed or diastatic skull fracture.
- Pneumocephalus.
- Cerebral edema.

11.7.4   MANAGEMENT OF MODERATE BRAIN INJURY (GCS 9–12)

- Serial neurologic exams are essential, as 10–20% of these patients will deteriorate.

- CT head should be obtained and neurosurgery consulted.
- Consider Tranexamic acid (TXA) within 3 h of injury. TXA 1 g is infused over 10 min, followed by an intravenous (IV) infusion of 1 g over 8 h.[4]
- Patients should be admitted to an intensive care unit (ICU) or similar care area that can provide adequate neurologic checks for 12–24 h.
- Repeat CT head if there is an abnormality and deterioration of patient's neurologic status.
- Caution with the use of narcotics. Avoid hypercapnia. If patient cannot maintain their airway, urgent intubation may be necessary.
- If the patient deteriorates, manage as severe brain injury. If patient improves, may discharge after 24 h with follow-up in clinic.

11.7.5   MANAGEMENT OF SEVERE BRAIN INJURY (GCS 3–8)[13]

11.7.5.1   Ventilation Support

- Early intubation.
- Avoid hypoxia: maintain oxygen saturation >98%, PaO_2 >60 mmHg.
- Consider the use of end tidal CO_2 ($ETCO_2$) for all ventilated TBI patients.
- Avoid hyperventilation: reducing pCO_2 <30 mmHg can cause vasoconstriction leading to cerebral ischemia. Goal for pCO_2 is approximately 35 mmHg. A brief period of hyperventilation ($PaCO_2$ 25–30 mmHg) may be necessary in neurologic deterioration to lower ICP until other measures are introduced.
- Avoid hypercarbia (pCO_2 > 45 mmHg) because it causes vasodilation and increases intracranial pressure (ICP).
- Increased PEEP may increase ICP. PEEP above 10 mmHg should be used in conjunction with close monitoring of ICP.

11.7.5.2 Hemodynamic Management

- Intravenous fluids: Normal Saline is preferred. Avoid glucose-containing fluid to avoid hyperglycemia (maintain glucose at 140–180 mg/dl), or hypotonic fluid to avoid hyponatremia.
- Blood pressure goals: Maintain normovolemia and normotension.
  - SBP ≥100 mmHg for patients 50 to 69 years old.
  - SBP ≥110 mmHg for patients 15 to 49 or >70 years old.[14]
- Hypotension and hypoxia will double the mortality risk.
- Intracranial hemorrhage cannot cause hemorrhagic shock. If hypotension occurs, explore other causes.
- Neurologic exams are unreliable when the patient is hypotensive.

11.7.5.3 Cerebral Perfusion Pressure (CPP)

- One-third of TBI has disrupted cerebral autoregulation.
- Low CPP is associated with secondary brain injury.
- CPP = MAP – ICP, goal CPP 60–70 mmHg, MAP 80–100 mmHg.
- Hypertension can worsen cerebral edema; therefore, the initial focus should be on lowering ICP.

11.7.5.4 Anticonvulsants

- Intracranial hemorrhage is associated with an increased risk of early (first week) post-traumatic seizures, and prophylactic anticonvulsant therapy may be appropriate.
- Levetiracetam (Keppra): loading dose 20 mg/kg, maintenance dose 1 g Q12 H for 7 days.
- May consider phenytoin: loading dose 1 g IV and maintenance dose 100 mg/8h.
- EEG is indicated if there is persistent impaired consciousness that is disproportionate to the extent of injury; continue anti-seizure medication if there is evidence of convulsive activity.
- If seizures are not controlled, may use diazepam or lorazepam.
- Prolonged seizure (30–60 min) may cause secondary brain injury.

11.7.5.5 Imaging

- Head CT should be obtained as soon as possible but do not delay for transfer.
- Repeat CT within 24 h for neurologic changes or if initial head CT showed contusion or hematoma.
- Midline shift of 5 mm or greater is often an indication for surgical intervention.

11.7.5.6 VTE Prophylaxis

- SCDs are appropriate.
- Subcutaneous heparin, 5000 units TID or enoxaparin, 40 mg daily may be safe but should be initiated after consultation with Neurosurgery. Repeat brain CT should be obtained after this is begun.

11.7.5.7 Management of Coagulopathy (see Section 11.3.3)

- Tranexamic acid (TXA) 1 g is infused over 10 min, followed by an intravenous (IV) infusion of 1 g over 8 h.
- Obtain medication history of antiplatelet or anticoagulation medications and INR.
- Rapid reversal of anticoagulation should be performed.
- If on Coumadin, reverse with PCC and Vitamin K.
- If thrombocytopenic, transfuse platelets with a goal of >75,000.

11.7.6 IMPENDING CEREBRAL HERNIATION

11.7.6.1 Signs of Impending Cerebral Herniation

- Significant pupillary asymmetry
- Unilateral or bilateral fixed and dilated pupils
- Decorticate or decerebrate posturing
- Respiratory depression
- "Cushing's triad": hypertension, bradycardia, and irregular respiration

11.7.6.2 Treatment of Impending Cerebral Herniation (Temporizing Measures Until Neurosurgical Intervention)

- Endotracheal intubation.
- Elevation of the head of bed (more than 45°).
- Brief hyperventilation to a pCO$_2$ of approximately 30 mmHg (end-tidal carbon dioxide [ETCO$_2$] 25 to 30 mmHg).
- Hyperosmolar therapy (Section 11.8.5): options are (1) 3% hypertonic saline bolus, (2) 23.4 % hypertonic saline, and (3) mannitol – when making a selection, consider vascular access and what can be available/administered the fastest.
- 3% hypertonic saline bolus (250 ml) can be administered through peripheral access.
- 23.4% hypertonic saline, 30–60 ml/10 min rapid infusion can cause transient profound hypotension. This must be administered through central venous or intra-osseous access.
- Mannitol 20% (20 g in 100 ml) bolus 1–1.5 g/kg over 5 min. Mannitol is a potent osmotic diuretic and will worsen hypotension. Hypertonic saline is preferred.
- Maintain MAP 80 to 100 mmHg with fluid and vasopressors.

11.8 Intracranial Pressure (ICP) Management

- ICP is normally approximately 10 mmHg.
- Cerebral perfusion pressure (CPP) = Mean Arterial Pressure (MAP) – ICP.

11.8.1 INDICATION

- Consider when GCS ≤8 with abnormal CT (mass effect from lesions such as hematomas, contusions, or swelling).

or

• Normal CT scan if two of the following are present: age >40 years, motor posturing, or SBP <90 mmHg.

11.8.2   ICP MONITOR ONLY VERSUS EXTERNAL VENTRICULAR DRAIN (EVD) (TABLE 11.8)

Table 11.8 ICP monitor vs. EVD

ICP monitor ("bolt")	EVD
• Lower risk of hemorrhage and infection	• Most accurate and cost-effective to monitor ICP
• Easier to insert	• Therapeutic advantage to drain CSF if rises in ICP

11.8.3   CEREBROSPINAL FLUID DRAINAGE

• Drainage of CSF can be done to lower ICP when EVD is in place.
• Drainage may be continuous or intermittent. Guidelines recommend continuous CSF drainage for better control of ICP compared with intermittent drainage. Continuous drainage is recommended with a GCS score <6 in the first 12 h.[14,15]
• Caution must be utilized with continuous drainage. Excessive drainage can lead to ventricular collapse and malfunctioning or occlusion of the catheter in the setting of cerebral edema and small ventricles.

11.8.4   SEDATION AND ANALGESIA

• Lower ICP by reducing cerebral metabolic demand, CBF, and cerebral blood volume.

- Opioid analgesia is preferred to sedative infusion.
- Fentanyl is preferred over morphine (greater efficacy and minimized hemodynamic instability).
- Propofol is a preferred sedating agent (decreasing cerebral metabolic demand and ICP, short duration to allow intermittent clinical neurologic assessment). The propofol infusion syndrome (severe metabolic acidosis, rhabdomyolysis, hyperkalemia, renal failure, and cardiovascular collapse) is rare, usually with higher dose and extended time.
- If hypotension is due to sedation, consider fluids and vasopressors to maintain CPP goals.
- Neuromuscular blockade may decrease ICP elevations associated with ventilator dyssynchrony and coughing but should not be used as a routine measure.

11.8.5 OSMOTIC THERAPY

- Mannitol or Hypertonic Saline can be used to lessen cerebral edema after CSF drainage, analgesia, and sedation.
- 3% NaCl through central venous access (short term use via peripheral IV access while obtaining central access may be acceptable) to achieve a sodium goal of 145 to 155 mEq/l (trend Na every 6 h).
- Additional 30 ml bolus doses of 23.4% NaCl over 10 min to treat acute ICP elevations (must be administered per central venous or intraosseous device).
- Mannitol boluses of 0.25 to 1 g/kg every four to 6 h as needed. Trend osmolality every 6 h. Target osmolality 300–320 mOsm/l.
- Hypernatremia should be corrected gradually. Avoid correction by more than 5 mEq/l in a 24-h period.
- In elevated ICP or severe cerebral edema, may allow Na to rise 160 to 165 mEq/l.

11.8.6   REFRACTORY ICP ELEVATION

Decompressive craniectomy, barbiturate coma, or hypothermia may be options.

11.8.6.1   Decompressive Craniectomy

- TBI patients with ICP elevation refractory to medical therapy.
- A hemicraniectomy (for unilateral injury) or sometimes large bifrontal craniectomy (for bifrontal or diffuse injury).
- The middle cranial fossa should be adequately decompressed to minimize the risk of uncal herniation, which may occur despite normal ICP.
- Generous durotomy must be performed, since most of the reduction in ICP is achieved by opening the dura.

11.8.6.2   Barbiturate Coma

- Pentobarbital and thiopental infusions in elevated ICP refractory to other therapies.
- Effective for the control of ICP but not shown to improve outcomes.
- When first-line measures (hyperosmolar therapy, deep sedation) are ineffective and surgical decompression is not feasible.
- Continuous electroencephalography (EEG) monitoring is used, with the pentobarbital infusion titrated to produce a burst-suppression pattern.

11.8.6.3   Hypothermia

- Reduces ICP, is neuroprotective, and limits secondary brain injury.
- Effective for the control of ICP but has not been shown to improve outcomes.

11.8.7   MANAGEMENT OF DEVASTATING BRAIN INJURY (DBI)[16]

- DBI is defined as neurological injury where there is an immediate threat to life from neurologic cause, and comfort care is considered.
- Decision regarding withdrawal of care and determination of clinical response should be delayed for 72 h.
- Prognostication should not be based on a clinical scoring system but on individualized assessments of risk factors. In TBI, the following are associated with in hospital mortality: pupillary changes, extremes of age, low GCS, high injury severity score (ISS), need for intubation, hypoxia, hypotension, coagulopathy, transfusion, and spinal injury.
- Early, frequent, and consistent multidisciplinary communication should occur and include family/healthcare proxy and other resources (social services, palliative care).

11.9 Extremity Compartment Syndrome

- Diagnosis is based on clinical examination with emphasis on the evolution of the "5Ps:" Pain, Paresthesia, Poikilothermia, Paralysis, and Pulselessness.
- Loss of pulses is a late development of compartment syndrome.
- Compartment pressure measurement may aid in diagnosis but this is primarily a clinical assessment.
- Compartment pressure >30 mmHg, or mean arterial pressure – compartment pressure <30 mmHg strongly suggests the diagnosis.
- Immediate fasciotomy is indicated for definitive management.

11.10 Burn

In those unusual circumstances where neurotrauma is compounded by significant burn injury, the risks of hypotension and hypoxemia are increased. An estimate of burn size is critical in planning fluid resuscitation. Early intubation and positive pressure assistance is vital to avoid hypoxemia. For severe injury, consideration should be given to transfer to a burn center.

11.10.1 CLASSIFICATION

- **Superficial Burn** (example sunburn): involve only the epidermal layer with erythema, pain, no blisters.
- **Partial Thickness Burn** (superficial or deep): involves the epidermis and portions of the dermis with red or mottled appearance, swelling and blisters, and pain.
- **Full Thickness**: involves all layers of the dermis: usually dark and leathery, non-blanching, painless and dry, with eschar.

11.10.2 ESTIMATION OF BURN SIZE

Rules of Nines: calculate the body-surface area (BSA). This only applies to second and third-degree burns (Figure 11.2).

Another way to estimate burn size is to use the patient's palm. The size of the patient's palm is about 1% of the body.

11.10.3 CALCULATION OF FLUID INITIAL RESUSCITATION

- **Parkland Formula**: used to estimate fluid volume required (Lactated Ringers solution) for resuscitation: 4 ml × %BSA × weight (kg). Note that

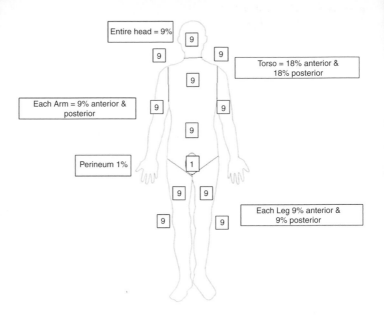

Figure 11.2 Rule of nines (burn percentage in adult)

this is based on the estimated amount of partial and full thickness burn only. Half of this volume is infused over the first 8 h from the time of the initial burn, and the second half is infused over the next 16 h. This calculated volume may be adjusted based on the patient's response (vital signs, urine output).

- **Modified Brooke Formula**: Total volume LR = 2 ml × %BSA × weight (kg).

11.10.4 TRANSFER CRITERIA TO BURN CENTER[17]

- Partial thickness burns greater than 10% total body surface area (TBSA).
- Burns that involve the face, hands, feet, genitalia, perineum, or major joints.

- Third-degree burns in any age group.
- Electrical burns, including lightning injury.
- Chemical burns.
- Inhalation injury.
- Burn injury in patients with preexisting medical disorders that could complicate management, prolong recovery, or affect mortality.
- Any patient with burns and concomitant trauma in which the burn injury poses the greatest risk of morbidity or mortality.
- Medical control plan and triage protocols.
- Burned children in hospitals without qualified personnel or equipment for the care of children.
- Burn injury in patients who will require special social, emotional, or rehabilitative intervention.

References

1. American College of Surgeons CoT. ATLS-Advance Trauma Life Support. 2019.
2. Patel MB, Humble SS, Cullinane DC, Day MA, Jawa RS, Devin CJ, et al. Cervical spine collar clearance in the obtunded adult blunt trauma patient: a systematic review and practice management guideline from the Eastern Association for the Surgery of Trauma. J Trauma Acute Care Surg. 2015;78(2):430–41.
3. Zuckerbraun BS, Peitzman AB, Billiar TR. Shock. In: Brunicardi FC, Andersen DK, Billiar TR, Dunn DL, Kao LS, Hunter JG, et al., eds. Schwartz's principles of surgery, 11th ed. New York: McGraw-Hill Education; 2019.
4. CRASH-3 Trial Collaborators. Effects of tranexamic acid on death, disability, vascular occlusive events and other morbidities in patients with acute traumatic brain injury (CRASH-3): a randomised, placebo-controlled trial. Lancet. 2019;394(10210):1713–23.
5. Surgical Education ORMC. Chest Tube Management. 2009.
6. Cothren Burlew C, Moore EE. Trauma. In: Brunicardi FC, Andersen DK, Billiar TR, Dunn DL, Kao LS, Hunter JG, et al., eds. Schwartz's principles of surgery, 11th ed. New York: McGraw-Hill Education; 2019.
7. Schein M, Ivatury R. Intra-abdominal hypertension and the abdominal compartment syndrome. Br J Surg. 1998;85(8):1027–28.

8. Stiell IG, Wells GA, Vandemheen K, Clement C, Lesiuk H, Laupacis A, et al. The Canadian CT Head Rule for patients with minor head injury. Lancet. 2001;357 (9266):1391–96.

9. Schuster R, Waxman K. Is repeated head computed tomography necessary for traumatic intracranial hemorrhage? Am Surgeon. 2005;71(9):701–04.

10. Joseph B, Aziz H, Pandit V, Kulvatunyou N, Hashmi A, Tang A, et al. A three-year prospective study of repeat head computed tomography in patients with traumatic brain injury. J Am Coll Surg. 2014;219(1):45–51.

11. Sifri ZC, Homnick AT, Vaynman A, Lavery R, Liao W, Mohr A, et al. A prospective evaluation of the value of repeat cranial computed tomography in patients with minimal head injury and an intracranial bleed. J Trauma. 2006;61(4):862–67.

12. Valadka AB. Traumatic brain injury. In: Moore EE, Feliciano DV, Mattox KL, eds. Trauma, 8th ed. New York: McGraw-Hill Education; 2017.

13. Hawryluk GWJ, Aguilera S, Buki A, Bulger E, Citerio G, Cooper DJ, et al. A management algorithm for patients with intracranial pressure monitoring: the Seattle International Severe Traumatic Brain Injury Consensus Conference (SIBICC). Intensive Care Med. 2019;45(12):1783–94.

14. Carney N, Totten AM, O'Reilly C, Ullman JS, Hawryluk GW, Bell MJ, et al. Guidelines for the management of severe traumatic brain injury, 4th ed. Neurosurgery. 2017;80 (1):6–15.

15. Nwachuku EL, Puccio AM, Fetzick A, Scruggs B, Chang YF, Shutter LA, et al. Intermittent versus continuous cerebrospinal fluid drainage management in adult severe traumatic brain injury: assessment of intracranial pressure burden. Neurocrit Care. 2014;20(1):49–53.

16. Souter MJ, Blissitt PA, Blosser S, Bonomo J, Greer D, Jichici D, et al. Recommendations for the critical care management of devastating brain injury: prognostication, psychosocial, and ethical management: a position statement for healthcare professionals from the neurocritical care society. Neurocrit Care. 2015;23(1):4–13.

17. American Burn Association. Burn Center Referral Criteria. Available from: http://ameriburn.org/wp-content/uploads/2017/05/burncenterreferralcriteria.pdf.

12

Critical Care Management before and after Open and Intravascular Procedures

Aimee Aysenne and Martha Robinson

Abstract

Neurosurgical patients often require care in the neurocritical care unit, and neurocritical care patients often need neurosurgical procedures. A multidisciplinary approach is beneficial for care of these patients. The neurointensivist must have a basic understanding of the indications, operative procedures, and complications of neurosurgical procedures. These include open craniotomies, transsphenoidal skull base surgery, bedside intracranial pressure monitoring, and an ever-expanding array of endovascular procedures. This chapter serves as an introduction to neurosurgical procedures that may be seen by a neurointensivist and a primer for postoperative expectations and management. Disease-specific considerations are included for neurovascular pathologies, operative trauma management, and metastatic tumors.

12.1 Craniotomies

Operative Interventions: Craniotomies are performed for a variety of neurosurgical indications (Figure 12.1). A skull defect exposes the dura mater and allows for exposure of the brain. The cortex may be incised as part of the procedure, in which case antiepileptic drugs should be given. Prophylactic

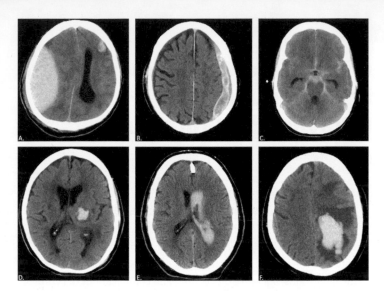

Figure 12.1 Subtypes of intracranial hemorrhage. (A) Epidural hematoma with contrecoup injury. (B) Acute-on-chronic subdural hematoma. (C) Subarachnoid hemorrhage. (D) Intraparenchymal hemorrhage. (E) Intraventricular hemorrhage. (F) Hemorrhage with underlying metastatic tumor

antibiotics are optional; when given, they are administered 30–60 min prior to the skin incision.[1]

Decompressive Hemicraniectomy: First-line for patients with ICP elevation due to focal compressive brain lesion.[1] Decompressive hemicraniectomy in stroke can improve morbidity and mortality following large ischemic infarct with malignant cerebral edema. Quality of life expectations should be established for patients greater than 60 years old.[1–3]

Suboccipital Hemicraniectomy: Approach is indicated to access the cerebellum, cerebellopontine angle, vertebral artery, fourth ventricle, posterior brain stem, or pineal region. Decompression is indicated for cerebral edema or hemorrhage in the posterior fossa or for Chiari malformations. Bulbar dysfunction or respiratory arrest may occur following the procedure.

Intubation for 24–48 h as a precaution is reasonable. In general, keep SBP ≤160 in the postoperative setting in order to avoid bleeding.[1,2]

Postoperative Care and Complications: In the postoperative setting, special care should be taken to ensure incisions are clean, dry, and intact, and any drains are working properly. The skull defect should be monitored closely; it should not appear tense or have drainage. Extra attention should be paid to protect the defect when patients are mobilized; patients should have a customized helmet when out of bed following hemicraniectomy. For immobilized patients, the occiput should be monitored routinely for skin breakdown; a foam head ring cushion can help to avoid such complications.[1,2]

Postoperative Deterioration: Emergency evaluation and treatment is indicated in a patient who declines postoperatively. Differential diagnosis should include hematoma (intracerebral hemorrhage, SDH, EDH), cerebral infarction (arterial or venous), postoperative seizure, acute hydrocephalus, pneumocephalus (tension or simple type), cerebral edema (brain may herniate through craniotomy and injure parenchyma on bone edges), persistent effect of anesthesia (especially paralytics), and vasospasm. Subdural or subgaleal fluid collections may necessitate drain placement. Air embolism should be on the differential if an open operation has interrupted the integrity of a noncollapsible vein. Focal extremity weakness in the immediate postoperative setting may be due to plexus or nerve injury incurred due to positioning during the operation.[1]

Postoperative Hemorrhage: Overall risk is 0.8–1.1%. Mortality of postoperative hemorrhage is 32%. Hematomas may occur at the site of surgery or in remote locations such as cerebellar hemorrhage after temporal and pterional craniotomies. Posterior fossa hematoma is of utmost urgency, as a small amount of mass effect can result in pressure to the brainstem or collapse of the fourth ventricle resulting in obstructive hydrocephalus.[1,2]

Postoperative CSF Leak/Fistula: CSF leak must be treated immediately. Etiologies can include poor wound closure, abnormal CSF flow dynamics, and subarachnoid scarring. CSF leak may exit through the skin incision, through the eustachian tube into the throat or through the nose, or through the ear in the case of a perforated tympanic membrane. Initial maneuvers to treat CSF leak include elevation of head of bed, placement of lumbar drain for CSF diversion, and reinforcement of incision. Should leak persist, become a CSF fistula, or result in a pseudomeningocele, operative intervention will likely be required.[1]

Postoperative Infection: Infections may occur superficially at site of wound or in the cranium. Cerebral abscess, subdural empyema, and osteomyelitis of the skull require surgical debridement and antibiotics.[1]

Postoperative Seizures: After structural lesions have been excluded with imaging, consider subsequent monitoring with EEG if a patient does not regain consciousness or has an unexplained neurological deficit. Standard medical treatment for seizures with benzodiazepines, antiepileptics, and possibly anesthetic agents are recommended.[1]

Postoperative Headache: Headache may occur in the immediate postoperative setting or present as a persistent headache.[1]

Syndrome of the Trephined: This syndrome may develop following hemicraniectomy. Patients may experience headaches, pulsatile pain at the site of the skull defect, insomnia, impaired concentration, and amnesia. Headaches have been attributed to tension on the dura and alteration of flow dynamics when the bone flap has not been replaced. Possible treatments include cranioplasty for large craniectomies, restoring function of the suboccipital musculature and/or temporalis, rigid fixation of bone flaps, meticulous efforts for tension-free closure of dura, and minimizing residual blood clot and bone dust during closure.[1]

12.2 Cranioplasty

Patients may incur skull defect following craniectomy or following significant trauma. Indications for cranioplasty include protection from future brain injury, relief of symptoms associated with syndrome of the trephined and cosmetic restoration of skull symmetry. Timing of the procedure should be tailored to individual patients. For open or contaminated wounds, it is reasonable to delay cranioplasty with synthetic materials for up to 6 months. Some skull defects can be repaired at time of fracture. For those skull defects that are not contaminated or performed emergently for cerebral edema, immediate cranioplasty is indicated.[1]

Operative Interventions: Patient's bone may be used for cranioplasty if it was previously extracted in a sterile fashion and was maintained in a sterile manner until the time of cranioplasty. Bone flaps may be stored via refrigeration. Storing of bone flap in an abdominal pocket is out of favor. Methylmethacrylate or mesh may be modified by the surgeon during the procedure in order to close the skull defect. Multiple commercial vendors offer prefabricated custom flaps that are created based from computer models of the skull defect; materials for custom flaps include methylmethacrylate, poly-ether-ether-ketone (PEEK), or titanium. Split thickness calvaria grafts are another option.[1]

Postoperative Care and Complications: Postoperative complications including hemorrhage, wound breakdown, or infection are similar to risk associated with craniotomy. Additionally, fluid collections or blood may also accumulate beneath the flap or between the skull and the flap, providing the most frequent complication.[1]

12.3 Transsphenoidal Surgery

Performed to access the skull base, including the pituitary gland, clinoid, and optic chiasm. Pituitary tumors comprise approximately 15% of brain tumors. Headaches, vomiting, and vision changes including field defects, decreased visual acuity, decreased color vision, and diplopia may develop. Surgical resection is required for the majority of pituitary tumors. For larger tumors, particularly craniopharyngeomas, a transcranial approach with craniotomy is often required. Prolactinomas may be managed medically with dopamine agonists. Preoperative planning includes assessment of pituitary hormone function. Nonsecreting tumors are typically not identified until symptoms present due to mass effect.[1]

Operative Interventions: The procedure is performed with endoscopy and microscopic dissection, often as a joint procedure with neurosurgery and oto-laryngology. Closure of the osseous defect in transsphenoidal and skull base surgeries may require gel foam, autologous transplants (bone, fascia, or fat), direct suturing, muco-periosteal flap, fibrin glue, or a combination of materials.[1]

Postoperative Care and Complications: Cranial nerve injuries, especially vision loss, damage to local cerebral vasculature, hydrocephalus, and change in status of pituitary hormone function, may occur. General hypopituitarism or central diabetes insipidus may occur; accordingly, urinary output should be accurately recorded in the postoperative setting. Patients should also be monitored closely for evidence of CSF leak. Sinus precautions should be maintained with no nose blowing, forcible spitting, heavy lifting, smoking, or use of straws. Sneezing should be performed with mouth open. Patient should not be submerged in water or go swimming until fully healed.[1]

12.4 Endovascular Neuroangiography

Angiography is the gold standard for cerebral vascular imaging. Therapeutic interventions are continuously evolving and expanding (Figure 12.2). As with any operative process, angiography is safest when performed in a repetitive, methodical, and consistent fashion.[4]

Preoperative Considerations: Patient's medical and surgical history should be reviewed thoroughly in order to identify any potential variants in anatomy or items that would require customization of the procedure. Contrast load and exposure to radiation should be minimized; steps taken to this effect can include using lowest-strength or diluted contrast, avoiding repeated injections, and aspirating remaining contrast from the catheter after runs are completed. All tubes and lines should be thoroughly inspected prior to angiography to remove any evidence of air bubbles, thus minimizing risk of air embolization.[4]

Premedication for Contrast Allergy: Patients with a history of anaphylaxis with exposure to contrast have a 17–35% chance of similar reaction on

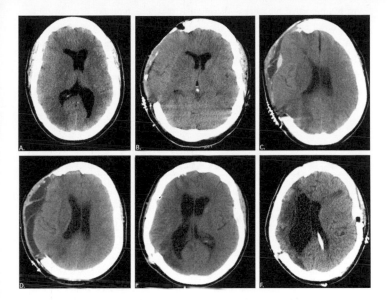

Figure 12.2 Right MCA stroke in patient with fibromuscular dysplasia. (A) CT Cerebral perfusion with RAPID software demonstrating core-to-penumbra ratio favorable for endovascular intervention. (B) Decreased right MCA flow per 3D vessel reconstruction. (C) Increased MTT and Tmax and decreased CBF in MCA territory with relatively preserved CBV. (D, E) "Flame-sign" of carotid dissection on CTA and dedicated angiogram

subsequent contrast administrations. Anesthesia should be made aware of allergy with advanced notice. Premedication should consist of corticosteroid and antihistamine administration.[4]

12.5 Post-Angiography Care and Complications

Reaction to Contrast Administration: Physiologic reactions including nausea, vomiting, headache, and vasovagal response can be managed with supportive measures. Allergic-like reactions typically occur within 20 min of contrast injection. Diphenhydramine should be administered for urticaria/erythema. Supplemental oxygen and beta-agonist inhaler (albuterol) should be administered for mild to moderate wheezing and bronchospasm. For symptomatic bradycardia, atropine may be required. Anaphylactoid reactions occur at an estimated incidence of 0.04% and require epinephrine administration.[4]

12.6 Vascular Access Site Issues

Groin Access Site: Following angiography, patients should lie flat, avoiding hip flexion, in order to lower risk of hematoma. Gentle reverse Trendelenburg is acceptable. Patients with manual groin pressure following angiography should be immobilized for at least 6 h. If the vascular access site is sufficiently above the bifurcation of the common femoral artery and a closure device is utilized (i.e. Angio-Seal™ or Mynx®), it is reasonable to reduce period of time patient is immobilized. Two hours at the minimum is recommended. Extended period of immobilization should be considered for those patients who have received tPA, antiplatelet, or anticoagulant agents. Limb immobilization device may be required in the setting of altered mental status or combative patient.[4]

Groin checks and distal pulse checks should be performed frequently. Doppler evaluation may be required; changes from preoperative intensity of pulses should prompt concern for possible distal thrombosis. Groin swelling should be concerning for hematoma or pseudoaneurysm. A pseudoaneurysm may form when the artery ruptures and extravascular hematoma is subsequently encapsulated; this may or may not result in narrowing of the lumen. Should this occur, apply manual pressure and continue immobilization. The sheath may be left in place when a patient has received multiple blood thinning agents or if a staged procedure is planned.[3,4]

Wrist Access Site: Radial artery access is advantageous in that there are fewer hemorrhagic complications and pseudoaneurysms but may be more difficult to access the cerebral vasculature.[4]

Blood Pressure Management: Postoperative blood pressure parameters should be at the discretion of the proceduralist. For procedures that include therapeutic intervention (thrombectomy, angioplasty, stenting, coiling, embolization, etc.), control of hypertension is of utmost importance; SBP <140 mmHg is a common goal. For diagnostic-only angiography, a goal of normotension is typically pursued. Long-acting antihypertensives should be avoided in the postoperative setting, as blood pressure fluctuations are common. Nicardipine is the preferred antihypertensive.[3,4]

Postoperative hypotension may be reflective of lingering effects of anesthesia, vasovagal reaction, dehydration, or contrast-reaction. For hypotension that does not resolve with sufficient IV fluid resuscitation, the possibility of retroperitoneal hematoma should be considered. CT of the abdomen and pelvis is diagnostic.[3,4]

Postcontrast Renal Considerations: Acute contrast-induced kidney injury is defined as an increase in baseline creatinine of 25% or more within 48 h of contrast administration. Patients with chronic kidney disease, heart failure, diabetes, and advanced age are most at risk. The injury is usually transient and results in long-term dialysis in <1% of patients. Adequate hydration before and after the procedure, particularly in those with established or borderline renal impairment, is key. Sodium bicarbonate infusion may be considered but remains controversial.[3,4]

Post-Angiography Neurologic Complications: Patients most at risk for neurologic complications are those with stroke or TIA, subarachnoid hemorrhage, greater than 50–70% stenosis of cerebral vasculature, advanced age (over 70), and prolonged angiograms. Re-bleeding of a recently ruptured aneurysm is the most severe neurologic complication; this is associated with a very high mortality rate. Microemboli consisting of dislodged atheromatous material or thrombus from the catheter and microbubbles are typically clinically silent, but should be points of concern in the patient with unanticipated postoperative neurologic changes.[3–6]

12.7 Intracranial Pressure and Cerebral Edema: Monitoring and Management

Intracranial hypertension is associated with many neurosurgical pathologies and interventions. Management includes measurement and treatment with invasive devices and pharmacologic agents. Osmotic agents including mannitol and hypertonic saline are standard treatment.[1–3,7,8]

Nonpharmacologic Considerations: Elevation of head of bed, avoidance of obstructing jugular veins by avoiding cervical collar and internal jugular catheterization, targeted temperature management, controlling pain and agitation, and minimizing increased intrathoracic or intraabdominal compartment pressures can maximize venous return. Hyperventilation should only be regarded as an emergency temporizing measure, for example, on the way to the operative suite.[2]

Invasive ICP Monitoring: Indications include cerebral edema, trauma-induced lesions (EDH, SDH, IPH, foreign body, depressed skull fracture), hydrocephalus, and severe TBI with an initial Glasgow Coma Scale score of ≤8. External ventricular drains are the gold standard for measuring ICP and are both diagnostic and therapeutic. EVDs can relieve pressure by draining CSF (Figure 12.3). The transducer must remain in line with the external auditory meatus for accurate monitoring and drainage. Fiber optic monitors can be placed in the intraparenchymal or subarachnoid space. Less frequently used are subdural and epidural monitors.[2,7,8]

12.8 Complications

Ventriculostomy-Related Infections: Most common complication associated with ICP monitors. At least one dose of antimicrobials prior to monitor insertion is recommended. The benefit of ongoing antimicrobials for prophylaxis is not well established. Antibiotic-impregnated EVD catheters have shown a trend towards decreased rates of VRI than with regular EVDs. Remove invasive monitoring as soon as clinically feasible to limit infections.

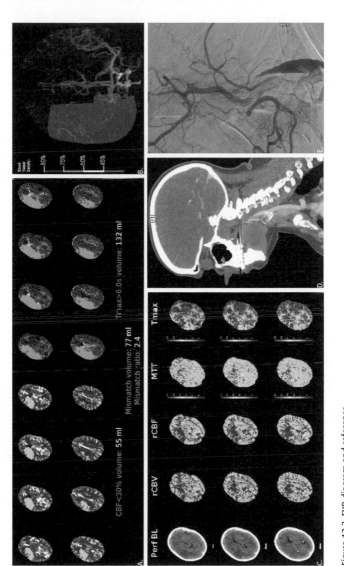

CBF <30% volume: 55 ml

Mismatch volume: 77 ml
Mismatch ratio: 2.4

Tmax>6.0s volume: 132 ml

Blood
Vessel
Density

—80%

—75%

—60%

—45%

B.

Perf BL   rCBV   rCBF   MTT   Tmax

C.

Figure 12.3 EVD diagram and reference

CSF sampling should be performed only when clinically indicated. Hospital-approved EVD management bundles help minimize infection rates.[7,8]

Hemorrhage: Reported rates of tract hemorrhages, extra-axial, and intraventricular hemorrhages vary. Patients with abnormal coagulation profiles have higher risk of hemorrhage; coagulopathies should be corrected prior to monitor placement if clinical severity permits. Timing of antiplatelet or anticoagulant therapies following EVD placement requires caution. Chemical VTE prophylaxis and sequential compression devices should be initiated as soon as possible.[7,8]

Malfunction/Obstruction: Neurologically injured patients may be confused or combative; care must be taken so that monitors are not dislodged. Bolt-connected EVDs may assist with preventing catheter manipulation. Pressurized irrigation bag should never be connected to EVD system. Initial beside evaluation of a poor or absent waveform includes ensuring there is still drainage from the system when the drain is lowered. Blood clots, infectious material, and local tissue may lead to catheter obstruction, and IVC may be dislodged from ventricle. These can better be evaluated with head CT. If the waveform is dampened, there may be air present in system; draining CSF should expel air. In some cases, this may be a normal finding (e.g. in the case of s/p decompressive hemicraniectomy, Figure 12.4).[1,7,8]

Other CSF Diversionary Procedures: First-line treatment for patients with ICP elevation due to acute hydrocephalus. Indications include SAH, IVH, IPH, shunt failure, brain tumor, and infections.[1]

Ventricular Shunts: Ventriculoperitoneal (VP) shunts are most common for chronic CSF diversion. Should patient require long-term alternate feeding source, recommend percutaneous gastrostomy tube placement be performed no sooner than 7 days following VP shunt in order to minimize risk of infection. Ventriculoatrial shunt (via SVC to atrium) and ventriculopleural shunts are rare, but satisfactory alternatives when indicated.[1]

Third Ventriculostomy: Endoscopic procedure for obstructive hydrocephalus.[1]

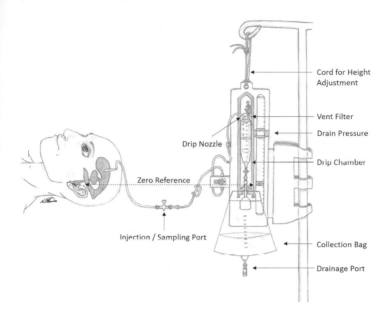

Figure 12.4 Right MCA territory stroke with malignant cerebral edema, evolving over time. (A) Cerebral edema with midline shift and loss of gray–white differentiation. (B) Status post hemicraniectomy with brain herniating through skull defect. (C, D) Adjacent fluid collection. (E) Status post cranioplasty. (F) Encephalomalacia approximately 1 year later with interval shunt placement for hydrocephalus

Lumbar Drain: May be used to reduce CSF pressure in setting of CSF fistula or CSF leak. May also be of use in testing for Normal Pressure Hydrocephalus.[1]

Ventricular Shunts: Shunt hardware consists of proximal catheter, reservoir, one-way valve, and distal catheter. Reservoir may be sampled to obtain CSF or to check ICP. Most modern valves contain magnets for ease of adjusting rate of flow. Make and model of shunt is identifiable based on radiographic appearance. Beyond failure of the shunt system, shunt infections are one of the most concerning complications. Most happen within 6 months of placement. Common source of infection is skin flora, wound infections, meningitis, or CSF pseudocysts.[1]

12.9 Disease-Specific Indications

12.9.1 ACUTE ISCHEMIC STROKE

Operative Interventions: Mechanical thrombectomy is indicated for select patients with a large vessel occlusion demonstrated on CT angiography. Indications include last known well time within 7.2 h and ASPECTS score greater than or equal to 6 on noncontrast head CT with significant neurological deficits as measured with the NIH Stroke Scale greater than or equal to 6. Extended time window may be used up to 24 h in patients with perfusion mismatch demonstrated with RAPID software in select cases.[3]

Postoperative Care and Complications: Care for the post thrombectomy patient is similar to other patients post endovascular procedures. There may be an increased risk of hemorrhage including groin hematomas and intracranially if the patient received intravenous thrombolysis. Blood pressure should be controlled. Monitor patients with neurological assessments and groin and pulse checks.[4]

12.9.2 CAROTID STENOSIS

Carotid artery atherosclerotic disease accounts for 10–20% of strokes. Rupture of atherosclerotic plaque can precipitate arterial thrombosis. Risk factors include smoking, hypertension, hyperlipidemia, and diabetes mellitus. Atherosclerosis tends to occur at vessel bifurcations and is accordingly common at the carotid bulbs, and the ICA and ECA origins.[3,5]

Operative Interventions: Patient with severe asymptomatic carotid artery stenosis with greater than 70% stenosis or with symptomatic carotid stenosis with transient ischemic attack (TIA) or ischemic stroke should undergo CEA or carotid stenting. Crescendo TIAs or watershed ischemic strokes are most at risk. The procedure should be performed within 2 weeks of the inciting event. Current data show long-term outcomes for CEA and carotid stenting are comparable. Specific considerations should be tailored to the individual patient.[5]

Carotid Endarterectomy: Open procedure with resection of the endothelium and atherosclerotic plaque from the wall of the carotid artery. Perioperative myocardial infarctions, cranial nerve injuries, and hematomas are more common than with endovascular approach.[5]

Carotid Artery Stenting: Endovascular procedure with stenting across atherosclerotic lesion to reduce risk of thrombosis and degree of stenosis. Carotid stenting is more effective than angioplasty alone and associated with fewer complications including restenosis. Stenting may be preferred in high-risk patients for general anesthesia, surgically inaccessible lesions, prior cervical radiotherapy, contralateral cranial nerve injury, contralateral carotid occlusion, prior CEA, or tandem occlusion. Carotid stenting is associated with a higher risk of perioperative stroke than CEA, but rates of stroke with stent placement have been decreasing over time.[4,5]

Tandem Lesion: Patients with carotid stenosis and acute ischemic stroke require endovascular clot retrieval and carotid artery stenting. Stents require dual antiplatelet agents and have a higher risk of bleeding.[4,5]

Intracranial Stenosis: Intracranial angioplasty and stenting is rarely performed after the results of the SAMMPRIS trial demonstrated superiority of medical management. It may be used in patients with refractory or recurrent symptoms.[3,4]

12.10 Postoperative Care and Complications

Perioperative Medications: Pre- and postprocedural dual antiplatelet therapy is recommended for carotid stents in addition to blood pressure control and statin. Up to 45% of patients have intermediate response to clopidogrel. Nonresponders to clopidogrel should be treated with alternate antiplatelet agents. P2Y12 level measures response; therapeutic window for clopidogrel is 95–208 Platelet Reactivity Units (PRU).[5] Above this level, platelet function is not properly inhibited; below this level, there is increased bleeding risk.

Ticagrelor may be an option. Statins have been shown to decrease rates of MI, stroke, and death.[3–5]

Hypotension and Bradycardia: Blood pressure may be labile within the first 24 h following the procedure due to changes in pressure at the carotid bulb affecting baroreceptors. Avoid long-acting agents that may affect blood pressure or heart rate. Titratable antihypertensive agents including nicardipine or clevidipine are recommended.[3]

Cranial Nerve Injury: Most common complication seen with CEA and is present in 8–10% of cases.[5] Hypoglossal nerve injury results in tongue deviation. If bilateral lesions occur, upper airway obstruction may result. Vagus nerve or recurrent laryngeal nerve injury results in unilateral vocal cord paralysis resulting in hoarseness. The mandibular branch of the facial nerve can also be affected.[3,5]

Neck Hematoma and Airway Monitoring: Hematoma is a rare complication of CEA. It is associated with risk of asphyxiation and stroke. Monitor for neck swelling, throat clearing, dysphagia, worsening hoarseness, tracheal deviation on exam or on X-ray, and air hunger. In the setting of imminent airway failure, wound should be opened and sterile-gloved finger should be used to evacuate hematoma prior to intubation and subsequent operative revision. Pseudoaneurysm can also cause neck swelling.[5]

In-Stent Thrombosis: For carotid stent placement, acute in-stent thrombosis occurs in less than 1% of patients within 24 h after procedure.[5] During the procedure, stent insertion may cause intimal injury, atheroma prolapse, or vessel kinking, which can result in in thrombus formation. Inadequate antiplatelet regimen, poor metabolic response to antiplatelet medications, and hypercoagulable state are associated with higher risk of thrombosis following a successful procedure.[4,5]

Vessel Restenosis: Restenosis rates following CEA range from 10–25%. Repeat CEA is associated with higher risk of stroke and cranial nerve injury than the initial intervention; stenting may be indicated in such scenarios. Restenosis following carotid artery stent placement within the first 2 years is more likely due to fibrous hyperplasia; after 2 years, atherosclerosis is the primary contributor.[4,5]

Perioperative Stroke or TIA: May occur as a result of embolic phenomenon, hemodynamic fluctuations, vessel dissection, or hemorrhage from reperfusion injury.[5]

12.11 Arterial Dissections

Cervical or intracranial arterial dissections can occur in the carotid or vertebral arteries. Stroke is the most common presenting symptom. Neck pain or headache may be present. Additional associated symptoms include Horner syndrome, lower cranial nerve palsy, pulsatile tinnitus, and cervical nerve root dysfunction. There is no inciting trauma in 60% of cases; however, mechanical triggers and minor head and neck trauma are common. Some associations are chiropractic maneuvers, wrestling, violent coughing, and simple neck turning. There are also reported cases of preceding infection prior to dissection. Spontaneous dissections are associated with fibromuscular dysplasia, Ehlers-Danlos, Marfan syndrome, Takayasu's disease, syphilitic arteritis, autosomal dominant polycystic kidney disease, Moyamoya disease, and homocystinuria. Genetic predispositions to dissection are rare in clinical practice.[6]

Literature is limited for IV thrombolysis and endovascular interventions with extracranial arterial dissections. Intravenous tPA is contraindicated for intracranial dissections. Classic "flame-sign" may be seen at the site of the occlusion on vessel imaging. Kidney function may be abnormal if the dissection extends to the level of the renal arteries.[6]

Operative Interventions: Endovascular treatments include extra- and intracranial angioplasty and stenting in addition to mechanical thrombectomy. There is a theoretical risk of false lumen perforation, but this has not been well established.[4,6]

Postoperative Care and Complications: Postoperative stroke prophylaxis should be initiated within 14 days of injury if possible. Cervical arterial dissections typically require antiplatelet versus anticoagulant therapy.

Direct oral anticoagulants are not recommended at this time, given the limited data on their use in dissection. Intracranial arterial dissections are at risk of subarachnoid hemorrhage, and anticoagulation should only be used with extreme caution.[6]

12.12 Extracranial-Intracranial Bypass

ECA-ICA bypass is an open operative intervention to improve intracranial perfusion. While most commonly used in moyamoya disease, such may be beneficial for tumors invading or encasing major arteries, aneurysms that are not amenable to direct clipping or to endovascular intervention, or severe atherosclerotic disease. Moyamoya disease is spontaneous, progressive stenosis of both ICAs due to intimal thickening with development of capillaries for a compensatory mechanism resembling a "puff of smoke." Juvenile forms of moyamoya are more likely to result in ischemic stroke and TIA, whereas adult forms are more likely to present with hemorrhage. Surgery decreases the future risk of stroke, increases the level of cerebral perfusion, and decreases the risk of death due to rebleeding in symptomatic moyamoya patients more than conservative treatment. Direct bypass surgery shows a significant benefit over indirect bypass surgery.[9]

Operative Interventions: Anastomosis between the donor vessel and cortical receptor arteries are used for direct revascularization. Indirect revascularization involves using connective tissue to cover the brain's surface; options include encephalomyosynangiosis, encephaloduroarteriosynangiosis, and omental transposition. Graph types include pedicled arterial grafts with the superficial temporal or occipital arteries, radial artery grafts, and saphenous vein grafts.[9]

Postoperative Care and Complications: Monitor for neurologic changes and CSF leaks; pursue tight blood pressure goals. Hypertension may cause bleeding at the site of anastomosis and hyperemia. Hypotension may lead to graft occlusion. Consider aspirin on postoperative day 1. Perioperative complications may include hyperperfusion syndrome, hemorrhagic lesions, ischemic insults, wound breakdown or infections, and perioperative death. Cerebral angiogram 2–6 months following the procedure is recommended.[9]

12.13 Vascular Malformations

Vascular malformations may be asymptomatic, incidentally identified on imaging, or symptomatic and may be congenital or acquired. Symptomatic malformations manifest with intracranial hemorrhage, seizures, headaches, or progressive focal neurologic deficit. Types of malformations include AVMs, anomalies of venous drainage including those involving the dura, cavernous malformations, and capillary telangiectasias. Hereditary hemorrhagic telangiectasia, an autosomal dominant genetic disorder, is the most common cause of brain vascular malformations.[1,10]

Arteriovenous Malformation: AVMs consist of a web of dysplastic arteries within the brain parenchyma that shunt directly into the venous system without an intervening capillary bed; the central-most tangle of vessels within the malformation is referred to as the nidus. Associated calcifications may be visualized on noncontrast CT. High flow rates are associated with shear stress, venous outflow obstruction, and arterial steal. Asymptomatic AVMs have a 2% risk of rupture per year. For AVMs that have previously demonstrated hemorrhage, the annual bleeding risk is 6% for the first year, then 4% yearly thereafter. AVMs with intra-nidal aneurysms and deep draining veins have a higher risk of bleeding; posterior fossa AVMs more frequently have associated aneurysms than supratentorial AVMs.[10]

Fistulae: Dural arteriovenous fistulae are direct arteriovenous connections that occur within the dura mater. If dural drainage from the fistula extends into a pressurized cortical vein, the resulting hemorrhage may appear similar to that seen due to venous sinus thrombosis. The baseline annual risk of hemorrhage is 3%; after initial hemorrhage, the annual rebleeding risk of such a fistula increases to 46%. Of note, there is a higher incidence of thrombogenic risk factors in patients with dural AVM than the general population.[1]

Cavernous Malformations: Cavernous malformations are low-flow assortments of dilated sinusoids lined by endothelium. Yearly hemorrhage rates are 0.4–0.6% per year, but become as high as 22.9% per year after an initial bleed has occurred. Resultant hemorrhages tend to be small in volume.[1]

Capillary Telangiectasis: Capillary telangiectasias may be associated with developmental venous anomalies or with cavernous malformations; they are angiographically occult and are common incidental findings at autopsy. They are often found in the pons.[1]

Operative Interventions: Treatment options for vascular malformations entail conservative management, stereotactic radiosurgery, endovascular embolization, surgical resection, or a combination of these modalities. SRS is generally performed for AVMs too high risk for resection; treatment leads to endothelial cell proliferation, vessel wall thickening, and eventually closure of the vessel lumen. The Spetzler-Martin grading system takes eloquence of adjacent brain, size of malformation, and presence or absence of deep draining veins into account in order to risk stratify AVMs for optimal management.[1,10]

Endovascular Procedures: CT and MR angiography may identify venous malformations, but digital subtraction angiography provides a definitive diagnosis and the most complete and exact data regarding spatial and temporal hemodynamic flow and "angio-architecture." Early venous drainage visualized on angiography is a hallmark sign of AVM. Endovascular embolization may be staged and is most commonly adjunctive therapy prior to surgical resection or SRS. In select cases, endovascular embolization may be definitive therapy.[1,4,10]

Microsurgical Resection: Microsurgical resection via craniotomy is a common method of completely and safely eliminating AVMs. This may be performed in isolation, or after endovascular embolization to reduce intraoperative bleeding risk.[1,10]

Postoperative Care and Complications: Seizures are more likely to occur in supratentorial AVMs than with posterior fossa AVMs; a superficial venous drainage component is associated with a higher risk of seizures. The primary complications of endovascular embolization include thromboembolic stroke and hemorrhage. Aneurysm rupture is rare. Control of hypertension is imperative given the risks associated with changes in flow dynamics.[10]

12.14 Intraparenchymal Hemorrhage

Operative Interventions: EVD should be placed in patients with supratentorial IPH and decreased level of consciousness and/or radiographic evidence of hydrocephalus. Depending on size, location, and expansion of hematoma, patients may require hematoma evacuation or surgical decompression. Due to constraints of the posterior fossa, there should be a low threshold for hematoma evacuation and suboccipital decompression in patients with cerebellar hemorrhage.[7,11]

Postoperative Care and Complications: Prophylactic antiepileptic drugs should not be administered. AEDs should certainly be started in those patients demonstrating seizure; a high index of clinical suspicion for seizure in ICH patients with decreased level of consciousness should be maintained. Patients with venous sinus thrombosis and cavernous malformation are more likely to have seizures than other etiologies of IPH.[1,7,11]

12.15 Epidural Hematoma

Head trauma resulting in a temporoparietal skull fracture can injure the middle meningeal artery; arterial bleeding dissects the dura from the inner table of the skull, resulting in blood in the epidural space. EDH typically occurs in young adults and is rare under 2 years of age or over 60. Male to female predominance is 4:1. The classical presentation entails immediate loss of consciousness following trauma, then a lucid period, and finally altered mental status, hemiparesis, and ipsilateral pupillary dilation from uncal herniation. Patients may also present with nausea, vomiting, headache, seizure, and bradycardia. On noncontrasted head CT, EDH appears as a uniformly hyperdense, biconcave lesion between the skull and brain parenchyma; there is often associated mass effect. EDH does not cross suture lines. Risk factors for delayed EDH include precipitous lowering of ICP, rapid correction of shock, and coagulopathies. Posterior fossa EDH may occur as well, particularly in the setting of occipital skull fractures; tears in the dural sinuses are often identified.[1]

> **Operative Interventions**: EDH evacuation is indicated if the volume is greater than 30 cm3 regardless of GCS. Nonsurgical management should only be considered if all of the following criteria are met: Volume of EDH <30 cm3, thickness of hematoma <15 mm, midline shift <5 mm, GCS>8, and no focal neurologic deficits are present. Craniotomy rather than Burr hole placement may be necessary. Adequate hemostasis and tacking dura up to edges of craniotomy assist with preventing reaccumulation.[1]

> **Postoperative Care and Complications**: General complications of craniotomy can be anticipated. Additional bleeding may occur, particularly with antiplatelet or anticoagulant medications. Hydrocephalus may require shunting. Additionally, any brain injury incurred from compression prior to EDH evacuation is likely to be permanent.[1]

12.16 Subdural Hematoma

Hematoma appears crescentic or concave on CT Head and does cross suture lines; SDH may appear more heterogeneous than EDH. Risk factors and management are determined by how long the blood has been accumulating. On CT, acute hematoma appears hyperdense (days 1–3), subacute hematoma appears isodense (days 4–21), and chronic hematoma appears hypodense (between 3 weeks to 4 months). Patients with severe head trauma and low GCS on presentation have the worst prognosis. Age >65 is associated with higher mortality and lower functional survival than younger groups.[1]

Operative Interventions: For patients with minimal symptoms or pre-served neurologic function, it may be beneficial to reverse any anti-coagulants or antiplatelet agents patient has taken prior to operative intervention. Location, size, and acuity of hematoma are taken into consideration with surgical planning. Evacuation may be performed with burr holes and craniostomy or craniotomy.[1]

12.17 Postoperative Care and Complications

Drains: Subdural drain can be retained in place for 24–48 h postoperatively until output is minimal. This reduces rates for repeat surgical interventions. Drainage system should be closed. Ventriculostomy catheter or small Jackson-Pratt drain may be used. For JP drains, gentle suction may be applied to the bulb to promote drainage with a one-way valve. Maintaining adequate hydration and having the patient lie flat in bed for 24–48 h post-operatively may promote drainage as well. Prophylactic antibiotics may be given from time of drain placement to 24–48 h following drain removal. CT Head following drain removal may be helpful to establish a baseline in case of subsequent clinical deterioration. There is higher risk of intracranial hemorrhage which may require additional surgery should hematoma recol-lect, and there is a risk of hydrocephalus. Additional concerns are failure of the brain to reexpand, reaccumulation of fluid in the subdural space, sub-dural empyema, and tension pneumocephalus.[1]

Antiepileptic Agents: Seizures including intractable status epilepticus may occur. Postoperative seizures occur in up to 9% of patients. It is reasonable to initiate seizure prophylaxis for up to 7 days following evacuation.[1]

12.18 Metastatic Brain Tumors

Lung, breast, and melanoma primary tumors precede the majority of metastatic tumors identified. Management of solid metastatic brain tumors is typically multimodal and may include chemotherapy, stereotactic radiosurgery, whole brain radiation therapy, surgical resection or debulking, steroids, and prophylactic anticonvulsants. Patients receiving steroids for tumor should receive a 50% larger dose 6 h prior to the OR. Multi-disciplinary team discussion and planning should be utilized to customize the treatment plan to the individual patient.[1,12]

> **Operative Interventions**: Patients with a favorable performance status, limited extracranial disease, and a single, newly diagnosed metastatic brain tumor should undergo surgical resection in addition to whole-brain radiation therapy as first-line treatment; this approach is superior to WBRT alone. Patients are excluded if there are radiosensitive tumor histologies or leptomeningeal metastatic disease.[1,12]

References

1. Greenberg MS. *Handbook of neurosurgery*, 7th ed. New York: Thieme; 2010.
2. Koenig MA. Cerebral edema and elevated intracranial pressure. *Continuum*. 2010;24 (6):1588–602. doi:10.1212/con.0000000000000665.
3. Powers WJ, Rabinstein AA, Ackerson T, et al. Guidelines for the early management of patients with acute ischemic stroke: 2019 update to the 2018 guidelines for the early management of acute ischemic stroke: a guideline for healthcare professionals from the American Heart Association/American Stroke Association. *Stroke*. 2019;50 (12):344–418. doi:10.1161/str.0000000000000211.
4. Morris P. *Practical neuroangiography*, 3rd ed. Philadelphia: Wolters Kluwer Lippincott Williams & Wilkins; 2013.
5. Lamanna A, Maingard J, Barras CD, et al. Carotid artery stenting: current state of evidence and future directions. *Acta Neurol Scand*. 2019;139:318–33. doi:10.1111/ane.13062.

6. Engelter ST, Traenka CT, Lyrer PT. Dissection of cervical and cerebral arteries. *Curr Neurol Neurosci Rep.* 2017;17(59). doi:10.1007/s11910-017-0769-3.

7. Fried HI, Nathan BR, Rowe AS, et al. The insertion and management of external ventricular drains: an evidence-based consensus statement. *Neurocrit Care.* 2016;24 (1):61–81. doi:10.1007/s12028-015-0224-8.

8. Tavakoli S, Peitz G, Ares W, Hafeez S, Grandhi R. Complications of invasive intracranial pressure monitoring devices in neurocritical care. *Neurosurg Focus.* 2017;43(5). doi:10.3171/2017.8.focus17450.

9. Li Q, Gao Y, Xin W, et al. Meta-analysis of prognosis of different treatments for symptomatic moyamoya disease. *World Neurosurg.* 2019;127:354–61. doi:10.1016/j. wneu.2019.04.062.

10. Derdeyn CP, Zipfel GJ, Albuquerque FC, et al. Management of brain arteriovenous malformations: a scientific statement for healthcare professionals from the American Heart Association/American Stroke Association. *Stroke.* 2017;48(8):200–24. doi: 10.1161/str.0000000000000134.

11. Gross BA, Jankowitz BT, Friedlander RM. Cerebral intraparenchymal hemorrhage. *JAMA.* 2019;321(13):1295–303. doi:10.1001/jama.2019.2413.

12. Nahed BV, Alvarez-Breckenridge C, Brastianos PK, et al. Congress of neurological surgeons systematic review and evidence-based practice guidelines on the role of surgery in the management of adults with metastatic brain tumors. *Neurosurgery.* 2019;84(3):152–55. doi:10.1093/neuros/nyy542.

13

Shared Decision-Making in the Neuro-ICU

Kelsey Goostrey and Susanne Muehlschlegel

Abstract

Shared decision-making (SDM) is a process involving clinicians, patients, and surrogates that is grounded in making treatment decisions based on the best available scientific evidence and patient's values, goals, and preferences. This collaborative style of decision-making is urgently needed in the Neuro-ICU to meet the existing deficiencies in clinician–family communication and decision-making. SDM conceptual models include the Ottawa Decision Support Framework (ODSF) and Interprofessional Shared Decision-Making Model (IP-SDM) and form the basis of decision aids (DAs), which are SDM tools. The goal of SDM is to increase patient-value congruent decision-making, improve the quality of communication between clinicians and patient/surrogates, reduce decisional conflict and passivity, increase knowledge of decisions, and promote realistic expectations of treatments and outcomes. Further research is needed and currently underway to establish the efficacy of SDM in the Neuro-ICU on family, clinician, patient, and healthcare utilization outcomes.

13.1 Introduction

Shared decision-making (SDM) is a process involving clinicians, patients, and surrogate decision-makers ("surrogates") that is grounded in making treatment decisions based on the best available scientific evidence and patient's values, goals, and preferences.[1] This patient-centered, collaborative process is a transition away from making decisions in isolation or using a traditionally physician-driven approach. SDM has become a highlighted topic in medicine after the strong recommendation for patient-centered care by the Institute of Medicine's 2001 report "Crossing the Quality Chasm" and the 2010 Affordable Care Act.[2,3] To increase and implement SDM in clinical practice, multiple studies have aimed to understand stakeholders' needs, identify barriers and facilitators, create SDM tools to meet these needs and assess the tools' efficacy and ultimately implement SDM. These studies have demonstrated that SDM has the potential to reduce decisional conflict and passivity, increase knowledge and readiness about decisions, and promote realistic expectations of treatments and outcomes.[4]

This chapter's purpose is to raise awareness of SDM opportunities and ongoing research efforts in the Neuro-ICU. SDM tools, such as decision aids (DAs), offer the hope to improve the quality of communication between clinicians and patients/surrogates; ultimately facilitating patient-value congruent care. The following sections of this chapter will outline SDM models and essential elements, the creation and implementation of DAs, perceived and potential barriers of SDM, and communication strategies to facilitate SDM.

13.2 Shared Decision-Making Opportunities in the Neuro-ICU

Existing literature suggests that clinicians are not adequately applying SDM principles and do not regularly elicit patient's values, goals, and preferences in treatment decisions through their surrogate decision-makers.[5] Research in the general ICU setting demonstrates deficiencies in clinicians sufficiently informing surrogates about their role, communicating long-term outcomes, and withdrawal of life-sustaining treatments as an option in an unbiased way. This is problematic, as several studies have found that higher levels of SDM are associated with greater family satisfaction and communication, reduction of decisional conflict and passivity, and more realistic expectations of prognosis.[4-6]

SDM and substituted judgment by surrogates are particularly important in the Neuro-ICU. This is because admitted patients generally lack decision-making capabilities due to the severity of their acute brain injury. Thus, decision-making responsibilities fall on surrogates, which can include a spouse, parents, children, or legally appointed healthcare proxies (HCP). SDM should be utilized in the Neuro-ICU when preference-sensitive treatment decisions arise or when defining goals of care.[1] An example of a preference-sensitive decision is whether to undergo a craniotomy for hematoma evacuation versus medical treatment in a patient with a large intracerebral hemorrhage. Defining goals of care is another instance wherein SDM can be utilized. Goals-of-care decisions require surrogates to choose between treatment options that will either prolong life or make their loved one comfortable via the withdrawal of life-sustaining treatments. Clinicians and surrogates must weigh many factors when using SDM in both instances. Challenges arise when patients neglect to disclose their values, goals, and preferences were they to suffer a devastating, life-threatening injury or disease. Even in instances when families openly express their preferences, the final treatment or goals-of-care decision can be muddled by psychological and emotional factors, surrogate and clinician projection bias, and level of surrogate health literacy.[1] SDM strives to ameliorate these complicating factors to help surrogates make patient-value congruent decisions, while also reducing decisional conflict and psychological distress. This style of practice shows respect for person and for the family unit.

The Ottawa Decision Support Framework (ODSF) and Interprofessional Shared Decision-Making Model (IP-SDM), discussed in the next section, are SDM frameworks clinicians can utilize to guide SDM in the Neuro-ICU.

13.2.1   SHARED DECISION-MAKING MODELS

There are numerous SDM frameworks and models used. The Ottawa
Decision Support Framework (ODSF) and Interprofessional Shared
Decision-Making Model (IP-SDM) are described here. Other models can
be referenced at https://decisionaid.ohri.ca/models.html.

13.2.1.1   Ottawa Decision Support Framework

Researchers at the Ottawa Hospital Research Institute developed the ODSF
(Figure 13.1) to help guide clinicians and patients to make informed health
decisions. This framework targets decisional conflict and is derived from
concepts and theories in general and social psychology, decision analysis,
decisional conflict, economics of expectations and values, social support, and
self-efficacy.[7] The ODSF is routinely used and highly efficacious. Over 30
patient decision aids (DAs) have been developed and evaluated using the
ODSF.[7]

The three principles of ODSF are decisional needs, decision support,
and decision quality.[7] These three steps are intended to help guide the
decision-making process by identifying patient/surrogate decision
support needs, tailoring decision support that meet these needs,
evaluating the quality of the decision, and assessing the outcomes of the
decision.[7] The assertion of the ODSF is that each step in the framework has
potential to influence the other. For example, decisional needs may affect
decision quality. If decision needs and decision support are unfulfilled,
this can affect actions and behaviors, as well as health outcomes,
emotions, and cost-effectiveness; ultimately, affecting the quality of the
decision. Clinicians may utilize the ODSF to foster informed, value-based
decisions that reduce inherent delay in decision-making, minimize regret
and blame, and maximize cost-effectiveness and efficiency.

13.2.1.2   Interprofessional SDM Model

Another SDM model developed and validated by the Ottawa Hospital
Research Institute is the Inter-professional Shared Decision-Making

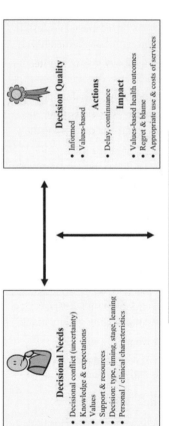

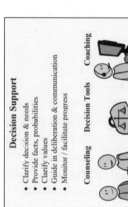

Decisional Needs
- Decisional conflict (uncertainty)
- Knowledge & expectations
- Values
- Support & resources
- Decision: type, timing, stage, leaning
- Personal / clinical characteristics

Decision Support
- Clarify decision & needs
- Provide facts, probabilities
- Clarify values
- Guide in deliberation & communication
- Monitor / facilitate progress

Counseling   Decision Tools   Coaching

Decision Quality
- Informed
- Values-based

Actions

Impact
- Delay, continuance
- Values-based health outcomes
- Regret & blame
- Appropriate use & costs of services

Figure 13.1 Ottawa decision support framework°

° Shown are the three principles addressing decisional conflict: decisional needs; decision quality, and decision support. These can be utilized to establish effective SDM dialogue.

From: O'Connor[7]

model (IP-SDM). An interprofessional team was utilized to design the IP-SDM, with the intention to expand SDM beyond the limited patient-practitioner dyad.[8] The IP-SDM model promotes a collaborative process between the patient, family members, and at least two healthcare professionals from different areas of practice. Figure 13.2 outlines the multi-actor and multi-step process of IP-SDM.[8] The top of the figure is the environment, which is representative of the three levels where the IP-SDM process takes place. These levels include social norms, organizational routines, and institutional standards. Under IP-SDM all three levels have potential to influence the decision-making process; therefore, elements such as cultural values and institutional structures must be accounted for when assessing and implementing SDM.[8]

The next level of the IP-SDM (Figure 13.2) represents the participants, or actors, involved in the SDM process; the patient and surrogates, in collaboration with the interprofessional team. In the IP-SDM framework, the interprofessional team is ideally made up of an initiator, decision coach, and an additional healthcare professional.[8] The purpose of a multi-disciplinary approach is to promote patient-centered care and informed, value-based decision-making.[9]

Following the establishment of SDM roles, the next step is for the initiator to indicate to the patient and surrogate that there is a decision to be made. It should be expressed that there are different options that can be applied to the decision, as well as recognition that equipoise exists.[8]

Once common knowledge and understanding of the decision and relevant options are achieved, the next step is information exchange.[8] It is important to note that starting in this level of the IP-SDM model, the vertical arrows indicate that SDM is an iterative process and that it is possible to revisit steps. Using evidence-based data, supplemented with SDM tools, the clinician(s) and patient/surrogate exchange information on the harms and benefits of each treatment option.[8] It may be useful to also include discussion on affective and emotional aspects of the decision-making process.[9]

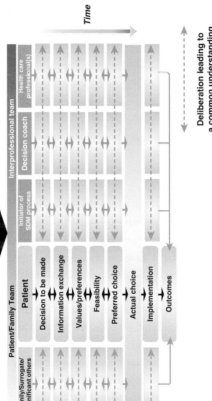

IP-SDM MODEL

Environment

Social norms · Organizational routines · Institutional structure

Figure 13.2 Inter-professional shared decision-making model (IP-SDM)[a]

[a]The double-sided vertical arrows represent the iterative process of SDM that can take place before making a final decision. The first two squares identify parties involved in SDM, while the subsequent represents achievement of equal understanding by each party. The dotted lines indicate discussion among those involved in the SDM process, as well as opportunity for further research.

From: Legare and Stacey[8]

The next step, which is discussion and clarification of values and preferences, may be done concurrently with information exchange.[8] In this step, if able, the patient is given the opportunity to express their values and preferences about the available options. If the patient is unable to participate, the surrogate will fulfill this role.

Feasibility of options is the next stage of IP-SDM. This takes into account the variability of resources (i.e. time and expertise), which may influence the decision-making process.[8] It would be harmful to promise a decision option to a patient/surrogate and later determine it isn't feasible. This could threaten the clinician-patient relationship and potentially increase decisional conflict. When feasibility is confirmed, the patient/surrogate presents their preferred choice to the clinical team. The clinical team may also offer its preferred choice as a recommendation.[8] Ideally, following collaborative discussion, all SDM participants agree on a decision. Practically, the patient and clinician are the only parties that need to agree on the final treatment decision.[8]

The subsequent step of IP-SDM is to implement the agreed-upon choice that best reflects the patient's values, goals, and preferences. There is also an opportunity in this step to evaluate implementation fidelity.[8] This may include assessing the quality of the decision and decision regret, if any. The purpose of this evaluation is to guide further decision-making.[8] Patients and their families may reassess and revisit outcomes if their first choice does not meet their expectations, which further demonstrates the iterative process of SDM.

Overall, the IP-SDM is a valid model that clinicians may use to guide implementation of SDM into standard clinical practice. Important considerations include the necessary time investment and iterative nature of SDM. However, time dedicated to this process has potential to reduce decisional conflict and passivity, increase knowledge about decisions, and promote realistic expectations of treatments and outcomes.[4]

13.3 Decision Aids as Shared Decision-Making Tools

13.3.1   WHAT IS A DECISION AID?

A decision aid (DA) is an SDM tool that is utilized to help patients and surrogates make difficult treatment decisions by providing objective information about available treatment options, including the harms and benefits of each.[4] The choice to do nothing is included as an option in DAs. Major professional critical care societies recommend SDM using DAs to reduce decisional conflict and surrogate decisions that are incongruent with patient values and preferences.[1,10] The International Patient Decision Aid Standards criteria (IPDAS) outline 12 dimensions that a high-quality DA should contain. Some of these dimensions include using a systematic development process, presenting probabilities, and establishing the effectiveness.[11] The full list is shown in Table 13.1.

13.3.2   EFFECTS OF DECISION AIDS ON DECISION-MAKING

To affirm the usefulness and efficacy of DAs in helping patients and surrogates make informed decisions on screening and treatment options, several studies have been conducted to assess various outcomes. The Cochrane review regularly evaluates and summarizes all existing DAs insofar as how they affect different decision-making and treatment outcomes.[12] The most recent Cochrane review (2017) found that DAs improve the knowledge of treatment and decision options and outcomes. This leads patients and surrogates to have more realistic expectations. It also found that DAs have potential to ease the burden of the decision-making process by helping match patient values with

Table 13.1 International patient decision aid standards criteria[a]

The 12 dimensions of the IPDAS checklist for the development of decision aids

1) Using a Systematic Development Process
2) Providing Information about Options
3) Presenting Probabilities
4) Clarifying and Expressing Values
5) Using Personal Stories
6) Guiding/Coaching In Deliberation and Communication
7) Disclosing Conflicts of Interest
8) Delivering Decision Aids on the Internet
9) Balancing the Presentation of Information and Options
10) Addressing Health Literacy
11) Basing Information On Comprehensive, Critically Appraised, and Up-To-Date Syntheses Of the Scientific Evidence
12) Establishing the Effectiveness

[a] A high-quality DA will meet the majority if not all the IPDAS criteria, which focus on the quality of content, development process, and effectiveness.
From: Elwyn et al. [11]

treatment choices, reduce decisional conflict and passivity, and ultimately make a decision.[12]

The Cochrane review also found that DAs do not improve patient adherence to treatment and only have a modest impact on treatment decisions. There is also only a slight effect on the DA group when selecting minor elective surgeries. However, participants in the DA arm of studies chose a major elective surgery less often than the usual care group.[12]

13.3.3 GENERAL RESEARCH OVERVIEW

While other areas of medicine have adapted DAs into standard care, this is not the case in the Neuro-ICU. The few DAs developed for use in the

Neuro-ICU are still in the development or feasibility testing phases; their efficacy has not yet been established. Studies in the medical and surgical ICU have demonstrated the need for SDM in this patient and family population. One study analyzed 71 audio-recorded goals of care family meetings with physicians and surrogates and performed a qualitative analysis. The study found that approximately one-third of the family meetings did not include any discussion of the patient's values, goals, and preferences when reviewing treatment options.[13]

In response to these findings, research has since been conducted to develop and implement SDM in the medical and surgical ICU. In 2012, Cox et al. developed a basic and preliminary paper-based DA for surrogates of patients with prolonged mechanical ventilation in the medical and surgical ICU. The DA was feasible for use in the ICU, and the overwhelming majority of surrogates and physicians felt that the DA was useful.[6] Its preliminary findings suggested an improvement in prognostic concordance between physicians and surrogates, improved quality of communication, and improved knowledge and comprehension of medical information.[6]

After this DA was successfully converted to a web-based digital DA, a multicenter efficacy trial was performed. The web-based digital DA included patient personalized prognostic estimates, explained treatment options, and patient-value clarification to inform a family meeting.[5] The primary outcome was surrogate-physician prognostic concordance at 1 year. Additional secondary outcomes included surrogates' decisional conflict, anxiety and depression, and quality of communication.[5] Unfortunately, the DA intervention had no effect on many of the study's outcome measures, including the primary outcome. Decisional conflict was the only outcome for which the DA intervention showed greater reduction compared to usual care ($p=0.041$; 95% CI 0.0–0.7).[5] Interestingly, physicians only integrated the DA in the goals of care family meeting in one-third of cases. This study also revealed the unique cognitive and affective challenges that exist for surrogates when making goals of care decisions that may have contributed to lack of intervention effect. Two potential factors that may have reduced the effect of the DA are (1) surrogate projection and (2) optimistic biases; only 43% of intervention surrogates "favored a treatment option that was more aggressive than their report of patient preferences."[5] Other studies have reinforced the presence of optimistic bias in surrogate decision-makers, which demonstrates the need for SDM in the ICU setting.[14,15] This also calls attention to the difficulty of effective communication in the setting of life and death decisions, and how it can often lead surrogates to select the default choice of full life support.[5]

13.3.3.1 Research in the Neuro-ICU

Currently, no DAs exist for any decisions in the Neuro-ICU, including the goals of care decision. This is problematic due to the alarming variability in rates of withdrawal-of-life-sustaining treatments across stroke and trauma centers.[4] To fill the gap in the Neuro-ICU, research funded by the National Institutes of Health is underway to create three Neuro-ICU-specific DAs for goals of care decisions in critically ill traumatic brain injury, acute ischemic stroke, and intracerebral hemorrhage patients.[16] Muehlschlegel et al. underwent a rigorous four-stage development of a DA for critically ill traumatic brain injury patients that meets international DA guidelines.[16] The vast majority of surrogate participants found the DA easy to use and reported it was acceptable for use in the Neuro-ICU.[16] Additional, similar DAs have been developed for intracerebral hemorrhage and large acute hemispheric ischemic stroke. Feasibility trial testing is underway in preparation for a multicenter efficacy trial; however, the results will take several years.

SDM may be an effective strategy for clinicians in the Neuro-ICU to help reduce surrogate decisional conflict and help make treatment decisions that are in alignment with patient's values, goals, and preferences, and DAs have the potential to help clinicians and surrogates appropriately navigate this decision-making process. However, further research on SDM and implementation of DAs in the

Neuro-ICU is needed, especially high-quality randomized controlled trials to show the efficacy of DAs on reducing decisional conflict and other outcomes.

13.4 Perceived and Observable Barriers of Shared Decision-Making

There are several perceived and observable barriers that can exist when trying to implement and use SDM, especially in the Neuro-ICU. One unavoidable challenge is the lack of a prior relationship between the clinician and patient/surrogate, which requires trust to be built before initiating SDM.[1] The clinician also must be willing to learn about the patient's values, goals, and preferences in order to guide the decision-making process. Another barrier surrounds the sudden nature of the illnesses that are typical of the Neuro-ICU; for example, a stroke or a traumatic brain injury, always occurring suddenly and unexpectedly, leaving families shocked and unprepared.[1] In cases such as these, it is important for clinicians to demonstrate empathy with surrogates, wherein they can employ the Ask-Tell-Ask method outlined in Table 13.2.[17] This method can help clinicians gauge if surrogates are ready to hear information about their loved one and if they are ready to begin participating is SDM.[1] Utilizing SDM has been shown to reduce surrogate distress and future decisional regret, therefore starting the process early could help combat this barrier.[4]

Another barrier that clinicians may experience is that surrogates may be unaware that there is a decision to make.[12] The underlying matter to this issue is that not all surrogates have the same medical literacy. Clinicians will need to guide their discussions based on the surrogate's competency and avoid medical jargon. One strategy to gauge a surrogate's understanding is to ask them how they will explain their conversations with the clinical team to other family members.[1] This is a nonthreatening way to ascertain a surrogate's health literacy and allows the clinician an opportunity to clarify misconceptions.[1]

Discomfort and inexperience with SDM are additional barriers that can exist for both the surrogate and the clinician.[12] The clinician can help guide the surrogate through the decision-making process by establishing trust, demonstrating empathy, and thoroughly explaining the surrogate's roles and responsibilities in SDM.[1] This would also be a good opportunity for the clinician to identify the extent that the surrogate wants to be involved in the decision-making process. Clinicians may also have discomfort and inexperience with SDM. In this case, it is important to not fall into traps of pessimism regarding the surrogate's ability to assume an active role.[12] Research has demonstrated that most surrogates want to share in the responsibility and burden of decision-making, and therefore should be given an opportunity to be involved in the SDM process.[1] Lack of training can be another concern for clinicians.[12]

Another barrier that can exist for both surrogates and clinicians is projection bias.[1] Despite the emphasis clinicians place on making a treatment decision that is aligned with the patient's values, goals, and preferences, surrogates can still project their own beliefs onto the decision-making process and exhibit optimistic bias.[14,15] This is demonstrated in a large trial where 43% of the surrogates randomized to receiving a DA to promote SDM, favored a treatment option that was more aggressive than their loved one's preferences.[5] One way clinicians can attempt to minimize this is by emphasizing to surrogate decision-makers that it is important to select the treatment option that is best for the patient, even if it isn't in line with their preferences.[8] Clinicians may also succumb to projection bias, particularly in the context where they do not believe that SDM is applicable to their patients.[1] Numerous studies have found that clinicians are not routinely utilizing SDM or eliciting patient or surrogate preferences in the decision-making process.[13] In this situation, clinicians must refocus and remember that they cannot transfer their own values onto patient treatment decisions. Rather, clinicians need to align themselves with the treatment option that matches their patient's values, goals, and preferences.

Some additional clinician barriers include time concerns and difficulty reconciling patient preferences.[12] Clinician time is valuable and scarce, but the potential benefits are a worthy tradeoff. SDM has shown to reduce decisional conflict and passivity, led to more realistic expectations of treatments and outcomes, minimized treatments that are misaligned with patient preferences, and diminished surrogate psychological distress.[4,5] Ongoing studies are assessing clinician time and burden as a secondary outcome.

An additional concern by clinicians about DAs is that they could bias patients and surrogates to choose less-expensive treatment options.[12]

Perhaps one of the most difficult barriers to navigate SDM in the Neuro-ICU is prognostic uncertainty. While several prognostication models exist for diseases of the Neuro-ICU, uncertainty always exists. Clinicians must emphasize uncertainty to surrogates when discussing treatment options and prognosis, especially as surrogates perceive prognosis with an optimistic bias.[14,15]

13.5 Communication Strategies: Do's and Don'ts

Considerable research has been performed to identify the need for SDM in the intensive care setting. White et al. have illustrated many deficiencies in physician-family communications and potential areas of improvement.[13,18] Despite this research, there is insufficient evidence to inform formal recommendations on how to communicate with surrogates. As referenced prior, the American College of Critical Care Medicine (ACCM) and American Thoracic Society (ATS) developed a conceptual road map that includes important facets to strengthen clinician-family communication and create a partnership with families when making treatment decisions.[1] However, until

Table 13.2 The Ask-Tell-Ask approach[a]

	Ask-Tell-Ask
Ask	Ask for permission to discuss prognosis
Tell	Convey the prognostic information
Ask	Assess the extent to which the patient/surrogate has understood the information

[a] The Ask-Tell-Ask approach can be utilized as a starting point to effectively explain a patient's medical condition and prognosis.
From: Buckman[17]

the efficacy of these communication strategies is empirically tested on family and patient outcomes, the following strategies should only be referenced as example language that may assist in beginning the SDM process.[1]

A prerequisite to starting SDM is to establish a partnership with the surrogate. The clinician should invest time early to build a strong rapport with the surrogate.[1] This could be accomplished through family meetings or inviting families to bedside rounds.

Next, it is important to provide emotional support to the surrogate and other family members. Evidence has shown that surrogate anxiety has been reduced and satisfaction increased when clinicians acknowledge emotions and demonstrate empathy.[19,20] Nurses, chaplains, or social workers can be utilized to provide additional support.[1]

Because surrogates will have varying levels of comprehension of their loved one's condition, the clinician should take time to assess the surrogate's level of understanding.[1] Once the level of surrogate comprehension is identified, information on the patient's medical condition and prognosis can be tailored accordingly. The Ask-Tell-Ask (Table 13.2) method may be utilized to help explain the patient's medical condition and prognosis to the surrogate decision-maker.[17] Some sample language for clinicians to use when exploring surrogates' understanding of the situation may be:

I know that you have already heard some information, and you probably have some understanding of your father's illness and just how sick he is. Before I start giving you more information, I would like to get a better sense of what you have been told and your impression of his condition. Can you please tell me what you understand about what is going on and how sick your father is?[1]

Next, the clinician should explore the level of involvement the surrogate decision-maker wants to have in the decision-making process. Following this discussion, the clinician should present all available treatment options to the surrogate decision-maker, including the risks and benefits of each option and the option to do nothing.[8] Clinicians should avoid medical jargon to maximize surrogate understanding. The next step is the exploration of the patient's values, goals, and preferences regarding the treatment options. Example language for clinicians to use is as follows:

We've talked a lot about your father's condition and the choices we need to make. Because different people make different choices, I need to understand what is important to your father. What makes his life worth living? Knowing him, do you think that he would want to go through these treatments if he would never be able to speak or understand anyone again?[1]

After confirming that the surrogate understands the patient's medical condition and prognosis, a pro-con deliberation should occur based on the patient's values, goals, and preferences. Utilizing SDM will promote an open dialogue setting to aid clinicians and surrogate decision-makers in making a joint, patient-preference sensitive decision; thus, equally sharing in responsibility and burden.[1]

13.6 Summary

This chapter outlined the principles of patient-centered care and SDM in the Neuro-ICU. It sought to provide a detailed overview on the process of identifying opportunities to utilize SDM and explaining SDM conceptual models and tools (i.e. DAs) in order to guide the implementation of SDM into standard care. SDM is urgently needed in the intensive care setting to meet the existing deficiencies in clinician–family communication and decision-making.[13] Greater exposure to SDM will reduce perceived barriers to implementation and increase the opportunity to improve the quality of communication between clinicians and patients/surrogates. Additional potential benefits of SDM include reduction of decisional conflict and passivity, increased knowledge of decisions, and promotion of realistic expectations of treatments and outcomes.[4-6] However, further research is needed and currently underway to establish the efficacy of SDM in the Neuro-ICU on family, clinician, patient, and health care utilization outcome.

References

1. Kon AA, et al. Shared decision making in ICUs: an American College of Critical Care Medicine and American Thoracic Society policy statement. Crit Care Med. 2016;44 (1):188–201.
2. Institute of Medicine (US) Committee on Quality of Health Care in America, In Crossing the quality chasm: a new health system for the 21st century. Washington, DC: National Academies Press; 2001.
3. Patient Protection and affordable care act. H.R. 3590. Public Law 111–148. 111th Congress. 2010.
4. Khan MW, Muehlschlegel S. Shared decision making in neurocritical care. Neurol Clin. 2017;35(4):825–34.
5. Cox CE, et al. Effects of a personalized web-based decision aid for surrogate decision makers of patients with prolonged mechanical ventilation: a randomized clinical trial. Ann Intern Med. 2019;170(5):285–97.
6. Cox CE, et al. Development and pilot testing of a decision aid for surrogates of patients with prolonged mechanical ventilation. Crit Care Med. 2012;40(8):2327–34.
7. O'Connor A. Ottawa decision support framework to address decisional conflict. 2006 [February 18, 2020]. Available from: https://decisionaid.ohri.ca/odsf.html.
8. Legare F, Stacey D, IP Team. IP-SDM model. 2010 [February 18, 2020]. Available from: https://decisionaid.ohri.ca/ip-sdm.html.
9. Legare F, et al. Validating a conceptual model for an inter-professional approach to shared decision making: a mixed methods study. J Eval Clin Pract. 2011;17(4):554–64.

10. Goostrey K, et al. *Adaptation of a traumatic brain injury goals-of-care decision aid for surrogate decision-makers to hemorrhagic and ischemic stroke with acceptability and usability testing.* Portland, OR: Society for Medical Decision Making; 2019.

11. Elwyn G, et al. Developing a quality criteria framework for patient decision aids: online international Delphi consensus process. BMJ. 2006;333(7565):417.

12. Stacey D, et al. Decision aids for people facing health treatment or screening decisions. Cochrane Database Syst Rev. 2014(1):CD001431.

13. White DB, et al. Toward shared decision making at the end of life in intensive care units: opportunities for improvement. Arch Intern Med. 2007;167(5):461–67.

14. Zier LS, et al. Surrogate decision makers' interpretation of prognostic information: a mixed-methods study. Ann Intern Med. 2012;156(5):360–66.

15. Lee Char SJ, et al. A randomized trial of two methods to disclose prognosis to surrogate decision makers in intensive care units. Am J Respir Crit Care Med. 2010;182(7):905–09.

16. Muehlschlegel S. Goals-of-care decision aid for critically ill TBI patients: development and feasibility testing. Neurology. 2020;95(2):e179–93.

17. Buckman R. How to break bad news: a guide for health care professionals, 1st ed. Baltimore, MD: John Hopkins University Press; 1992.

18. White DB, Curtis JR. Establishing an evidence base for physician-family communication and shared decision making in the intensive care unit. Crit Care Med. 2006;34(9):2500–1.

19. Fogarty LA, et al. Can 40 seconds of compassion reduce patient anxiety? J Clin Oncol. 1999;17(1):371–79.

20. Selph RB, et al. Empathy and life support decisions in intensive care units. J Gen Intern Med. 2008;23(9):1311–17.

14

Status Epilepticus and EEG Monitoring

Dionne E Swor and Deepika P McConnell

Abstract

Status epilepticus is a medical emergency that necessitates prompt recognition and treatment in order to prevent serious morbidity and mortality. This book chapter will discuss the pathophysiology, epidemiology, etiology, classification, management, and treatment of status epilepticus, refractory status epilepticus, and super-refractory status epilepticus within the adult intensive care unit (ICU) population. The chapter will then delve into continuous electroencephalography (EEG) monitoring in the ICU with an emphasis on the indication and duration of EEG monitoring as well as a brief discussion of the ictal-interictal continuum.

14.1 Status Epilepticus: Introduction

Status epilepticus is a medical emergency that necessitates prompt recognition and treatment in order to prevent serious morbidity and mortality. This chapter will discuss the pathophysiology, epidemiology, etiology, classification, management, and treatment of status epilepticus within the adult intensive care unit (ICU) population. The chapter will then delve into electroencephalography (EEG) monitoring in the ICU with an emphasis on the indication and duration of EEG monitoring, as well as a brief discussion of the ictal-interictal continuum.

14.1.1 STATUS EPILEPTICUS: DEFINITION AND PATHOPHYSIOLOGY

Several definitions exist for status epilepticus, in part due to the limited understanding of the pathophysiologic mechanism of this disease. This book chapter will take a simplified approach in delineating status epilepticus in terms of convulsive and nonconvulsive seizure activity. As such, we will use the most unifying definition of status epilepticus as proposed by the Neurocritical Care Society, which is 5 min or longer of continuous clinical and/or electrographic seizure activity or recurrent seizures without return to neurologic baseline between seizures.[1] This definition is based on the clinical observation that a typical seizure lasts fewer than 5 min and is self-limited, but seizures longer than 5 min tend not to end spontaneously.

The pathophysiology of status epilepticus is not completely known but is believed to begin at the molecular level with several changes occurring in unison, allowing a seizure to evolve and sustain as status epilepticus (Figure 14.1). This cascade of events promotes a hyperexcitable state while simultaneously downregulating inhibitory γ-aminobutyric acid (GABAA) receptors leading to the pharmacoresistence of GABAergic anti-epileptic medications, such as benzodiazepines, meant to treat and stop seizures.[2]

Prolonged status epilepticus (>20 min) can cause permanent neurologic injury, life-threatening systemic complications, and increased risk of mortality. Animal studies have demonstrated neuronal injury in association with both convulsive and nonconvulsive status epilepticus.[3] The cortex, thalamus, hippocampus, and cerebellum are particularly susceptible to seizure related CNS injury. The exact mechanism of neuronal injury is unknown but is felt to be related to excitotoxicity, apoptosis, necrosis, and mitochondrial dysfunction. Prolonged convulsive status epilepticus can induce a wide array of systemic complications, including changes in cardiac function, fluctuations in cerebral perfusion,

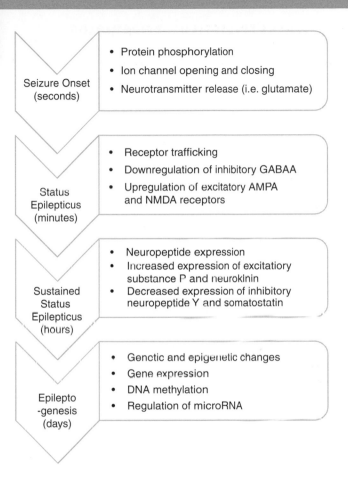

Figure 14.1 Pathophysiology of status epilepticus

decreased brain oxygenation, glycemic changes, ventilatory failure
leading to respiratory acidosis, and hyperthermia, rhabdomyolysis, and
lactic acidosis related to protracted muscle contraction.

14.1.2   STATUS EPILEPTICUS: EPIDEMIOLOGY

The annual incidence of status epilepticus is approximately 10–41 patients per 100,000 people. There is a bimodal peak in children less than 1 year of age and the elderly over 60 years of age, with an even distribution between males and females.[4] In the ICU seizures and status epilepticus can occur in up to 19% of patients; however, reports are varied, and studies are limited by their retrospective design and differing definitions of status epilepticus. Of the patients with diagnosed status epilepticus, 12–43% progress to refractory status epilepticus, and 10–15% progress to super-refractory status epilepticus.[5] The overall fatality of status epilepticus is approximately 15%, with greater incidence of fatality seen in elderly and patients with refractory status epilepticus.

14.1.3   STATUS EPILEPTICUS: ETIOLOGY

The International League against Epilepsy categorizes the etiology of status epilepticus into two groups: (1) known (symptomatic) and (2) unknown (cryptogenic) (Table 14.1). The symptomatic group is further subdivided into acute symptomatic, remote symptomatic, and progressive symptomatic.[6] Etiology of status epilepticus in the adult population is varied between studies and tends to fall within the acute symptomatic category with the most commonly reported causes being cerebral vascular disease, low anti-epileptic drug (AED) levels, and remote stroke.[5] The etiology of refractory status epilepticus is similar to that of non-refractory status epilepticus with the most common cause being low AED levels, followed by metabolic disturbances, and central nervous system (CNS) infections. The etiology of super-refractory status epilepticus is less well studied but appears to have a strong association with encephalitis. New-onset super refractory status epilepticus (NORSE) has recently been described in patients with new refractory status and no known history of epilepsy, structural lesion, or clear acute symptomatic cause. Within this

Table 14.1 Etiologies of status epilepticus

Known (Symptomatic)

Acute

Anoxic brain injury

Antibody-mediated

Autoimmune disorders

Paraneoplastic encephalitis

Cerebrovascular disease

Ischemic stroke

Intracranial hemorrhage (intracerebral, subdural, subarachnoid, and epidural)

Sinus venous thrombosis

Posterior reversible leukoencephalopathy

CNS Infections

Meningitis (bacterial, fungal, viral)

Cerebral toxoplasmosis

HIV-related diseases

Prion disease

Head trauma

Intoxication

Alcohol intoxication and withdrawal

Drugs intoxication and withdrawal

Metabolic disturbances

Acidosis

Electrolyte imbalance

Glucose imbalance

Organ failure (liver/kidney)

Pre-existing epilepsy

Breakthrough seizures

Withdrawal or low levels of antiepileptic drugs

Sepsis

Remote

Post-traumatic

Post-encephalitic

Post-stroke

Cortical dysplasia

Table 14.1 (cont.)

Progressive
Brain tumor
Dementia
Genetic disorders
Genetic progressive epilepsies
Metabolic disorders
Mitochondrial disease
Unknown (Cryptogenic)

population of patients, the most common etiologies of status epilepticus have been found to be autoimmune, paraneoplastic, and infectious.

14.1.4   STATUS EPILEPTICUS: CLASSIFICATION

Several classification schemes exist for status epilepticus based on semiology, etiology, and duration of seizures. For the purposes of this book chapter, we will use the Neurocritical Care Society's proposed status epilepticus classification, which divides status epilepticus into two categories: convulsive and nonconvulsive.[1]

1. Convulsive Status Epilepticus (CSE)
   a. CSE is defined as 5 min or more of continuous convulsive seizure activity or two or more discrete seizures between which there is incomplete recovery of consciousness.
   b. Characteristic clinical findings of CSE include:
      a. Generalized tonic–clonic movements of the extremities
      b. Mental status impairment
      c. Focal neurological deficits in the post-ictal period (i.e. Todd's paralysis)
2. Nonconvulsive Status Epilepticus (NCSE)
   a. NCSE is defined as electrographic seizure activity without clear clinical convulsive activity. Similar to the time frame for CSE the Neurocritical Care Society has also proposed a time frame of 5 min

or more of electrographic seizure activity or recurrent seizure activity without recovery between seizures for NCSE.

b. Characteristic clinical findings of NCSE include:

  a. Negative symptoms: anorexia, aphasia/mutism, amnesia, catatonia, coma, confusion, lethargy, and staring.

  b. Positive symptoms: agitation/aggression, automatisms, blinking, delirium, delusions, echolalia, facial twitching, perseveration, psychosis, and tremulousness.

c. EEG characteristics adapted from the Salzburg Criteria for diagnosis of NCSE.[5]

  a. Epileptic discharges >2.5 Hz lasting 10 seconds or more.

  b. Epileptic discharges ≤ 2.5 Hz or rhythmic delta/theta activity plus one of the following:

    i. Subtle clinical ictal phenomena during the above EEG patterns

    ii. Spatiotemporal evolution

    iii. EEG and clinical improvement after IV anti-epileptic drugs

Refractory status epilepticus (RSE) and super refractory status epilepticus (SRSE) are additional sub-classifications that are based on the response of status epilepticus to anti-epileptic drugs. Refractory status epilepticus refers to either clinical or electrographic seizures that persist despite adequate doses of initial benzodiazepine and an acceptable, appropriately dosed second-line anti-epileptic drug. Super refractory status epilepticus refers to seizure activity that recurs 24 h or more after the onset of third-line treatment with intravenous (IV) anesthetic therapy. Of note, the definitions of refractory and super refractory status epilepticus can apply to either convulsive or nonconvulsive status epilepticus.

One notable drawback of this classification system is that it does not account for focal status with retained awareness or epilepsia partialis continua (EPC), both of which may be seen in the ICU and require different treatment strategies based on the patient's clinical scenario.

14.1.5   STATUS EPILEPTICUS: DIAGNOSTIC WORK-UP

The diagnosis of status epilepticus involves a combination of clinical suspicion as well as laboratory tests, electroencephalography (EEG), and imaging.

1. Initial evaluation recommendations for all patients presenting with status epilepticus:
   a. Airway – Breathing – Circulation
   b. Fingerstick glucose
   c. Laboratory tests: CBC, CMP, calcium (total and ionized), magnesium, phosphorus, AED levels
   d. Imaging: non-contrast head CT
   e. EEG monitoring: continuous EEG monitoring if patient does not quickly return baseline or routine EEG if the patient quickly returns to baseline

2. Directed workup based on clinical presentation and patient history:
   a. MRI Brain with and without contrast
   b. Lumbar Puncture: CSF studies sent for cell count, protein, glucose, gram stain and bacterial culture, HSV 1&2 PCR, and fungal cultures
   c. Additional laboratory tests: comprehensive toxicology panel, ethanol level, ABG, LFTs, ammonia, lactic acid, urinalysis, urine culture, blood cultures, coagulation studies, β-HCG (in females), and creatinine kinase

3. Workup of cryptogenic super refractory status epilepticus or NORSE:
   a. Imaging considerations: CT chest/abdomen/pelvis, testicular and ovarian ultrasound or pelvic MRI to evaluate for teratoma, digital subtraction angiography (DSA) to evaluate for vasculitis
   b. Additional CSF studies: cytology, flow cytometry, viral PCRs, meningoencephalitis panel, and autoimmune/paraneoplastic panels
   c. Additional laboratory tests: microbiologic serologies, rheumatologic antibodies, paraneoplastic/autoimmune serology panels, heavy metals, porphyrins, and genetic testing

14.1.6 STATUS EPILEPTICUS: TREATMENT

The goal of treatment in status epilepticus is to gain seizure control as quickly and as safely as possible. Despite its recognition as a medical emergency, there are limited randomized controlled clinical trials available to guide treatment of status epilepticus, and the clinical trials that do exist focus on convulsive status epilepticus. As such, treatment algorithms published by the Neurocritical Care Society and American Epilepsy Society are based on the treatment of convulsive status epilepticus. There is no consensus regarding the treatment of non-convulsive status epilepticus, with recommendations of treatment based solely on expert opinion.

14.1.6.1 Treatment of Convulsive Status Epilepticus

Once convulsive status epilepticus has been recognized, stabilization of the patient, investigation of underlying etiology, and treatment should commence immediately and in parallel. Prompt treatment is crucial to minimize neuronal injury and to prevent refractory status epilepticus from occurring. Refer to Figure 14.2 for a summary of the convulsive status epilepticus algorithm and Table 14.2 for a detailed description and dosing of commonly used anti-epileptic drugs for status epilepticus. This treatment algorithm is a combination of the 2012 Neurocritical Care Society (NCS) and the 2016 American Epilepsy Society (AES) guidelines for the treatment of status epilepticus.[1,9]

1. First-Line Treatment: Initial Status Epilepticus
    a. After stabilization of the patient, if seizure activity persists for 5 min or more, the patient has met criteria for initial status epilepticus and should be given a benzodiazepine (either lorazepam or midazolam). This recommendation is based on the Veterans Cooperative Trial that compared intravenous (IV) lorazepam vs. IV diazepam + phenytoin, IV phenobarbital, and IV phenytoin for the treatment of convulsive status epilepticus. In this study, lorazepam was more

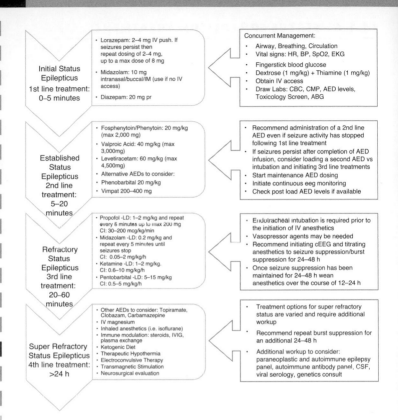

Figure 14.2 Convulsive status epilepticus algorithm[1,9]
Key: LD – loading dose, CI – continuous infusion

effective than phenytoin alone and was equivocal to phenobarbital and diazepam + phenytoin.[7]

b. If no IV access, then administer intramuscular (IM) midazolam. This recommendation is based on the Rapid Anticonvulsant Medication Prior to Arrival Trial (RAMPART) that compared pre-hospital administration of IM midazolam vs. IV lorazepam. This trial showed that patients who received IM midazolam prior to arriving in the emergency department were less likely to still be seizing and were less likely to require hospitalization.[8]

c. Diazepam has not performed as well as lorazepam to abort seizures in trials and carries a lower level of evidence than either lorazepam or midazolam.

d. Approximately 40% of patients with generalized convulsive status epilepticus will be refractory to first-line treatment and will meet criteria for established status epilepticus.

2. Second-Line Treatment: Established Status Epilepticus

a. If seizure activity persists following adequate treatment with a benzodiazepine then the patient has met criteria for established status epilepticus.

b. The Neurocritical Care Society 2012 guidelines for the treatment of status epilepticus and the American Epilepsy Society 2016 guidelines both recommend the use of phenytoin, valproic acid, or levetiracetam as second-line treatments for convulsive status epilepticus.[1,9] These guidelines are largely based on expert opinion as there was very little evidence to support one drug over the other at the time these guidelines were published.

c. The Established Status Epilepticus Treatment Trial is the first prospective randomized double-blind clinical trial designed to compare the efficacy of phenytoin (20 mg/kg), valproic acid (40 mg/kg), and levetiracetam (60 mg/kg) in the treatment of benzodiazepine-resistant status epilepticus. The results of this study were published in 2019 and revealed that there is no significant difference in the rate of seizure cessation or in safety between these three drugs.[10]

d. Alternate anti-epileptic medications to consider in this phase of treatment are phenobarbital and lacosamide. Both are mentioned in the NCS guideline but are not preferred agents as phenobarbital carries adverse side effects of cardio-pulmonary depression, and lacosamide has limited evidence supporting its use in treating status epilepticus.

3. Third Line Treatment: Refractory Status Epilepticus

 a. Refractory status epilepticus is defined as continued seizure activity following treatment with a first-line benzodiazepine as well as a second-line anti-epileptic agent.

 b. There is no clear evidence to guide treatment for seizures that continue into this phase. Expert opinion from the NCS and AES guidelines suggest either trialing a different second-line agent or proceeding with endotracheal intubation and initiation of anesthetic infusions.

 c. Recommended anesthetics include propofol, midazolam, ketamine, and pentobarbital (Table 14.2).

 d. IV anesthetics should be used in conjunction with continuous EEG monitoring with the goal of titrating the anesthetics to electrographic seizure suppression or burst suppression. There is no evidence supporting aggressive burst suppression over seizure suppression for resolution of status epilepticus, moreover, increased sedation requirements needed to maintain aggressive burst suppression has increased risk of adverse side effects.

 e. The duration of IV anesthetics after obtaining seizure control is unclear, with most experts recommending 24–48 h of seizure control prior to gradual weaning of IV anesthetics over the course of 12–24 h.

 f. Optimize anti-epileptic drugs by assuring adequate drug levels or adding AEDs to aid in continued seizure control during the weaning of anesthetic infusions.

4. Fourth-Line Treatment: Super Refractory Status Epilepticus

 a. Super refractory status epilepticus is defined as status epilepticus that continues or recurs 24 h or more after the onset of anesthetic therapy. It also includes recurrent status epilepticus during weaning or withdrawal of anesthetic therapies.[11]

 b. There are limited proven therapies for super refractory status epilepticus. Many experts recommend repeating a 24- to 48-h trial of

Table 14.2 Anti-epileptic drugs commonly used in the treatment of status epilepticus[1,9]

First-Line Treatment

Drug	Dose	Target Drug Monitoring	Adverse Effects	Clinical Pearls
Lorazepam	0.1 mg/kg IVP (max: 4 mg per dose)	N/A	Hypotension Respiratory depression	Max rate: 2 mg/min May repeat dose in 5–10 min
Diazepam	0.15 mg/kg IVP (max: 10 mg per dose)	N/A	Hypotension Respiratory depression	Max rate: 5 mg/min May repeat dose in 5 min
Midazolam	0.2 mg/kg IM/IVP (max: 10 mg per dose) Intranasally: 0.2 mg/kg Buccally: 0.5 mg/kg	N/A	Sedation Respiratory depression	Caution in patients with renal impairment due to accumulation of active metabolite

Second-Line Treatment

Drug	Dose	Target Drug Monitoring	Adverse Effects	Clinical Pearls
Phenytoin	LD: 20 mg/kg IVPB Maintenance: 4–6 mg/kg/day in 2–3 divided doses	Goal total trough level: 10–20 mcg/ml Goal free trough level: 1–2.5 mcg/ml	Hypotension Bradycardia Thrombophlebitis	Max infusion rate: 50 mg/min but can run slower to minimize hypotension To determine the need for additional phenytoin after initiation, check post load level 1 h after initial load is infused Administer through an antecubital vein or larger to avoid thrombophlebitis nd pain

Table 14.2 (cont.)

Second-Line Treatment

Drug	Dose	Target Drug Monitoring	Adverse Effects	Clinical Pearls
Fosphenytoin	LD: 20 mg/kg PE IVPB Maintenance: 4–6 mg/kg/day in 2–3 divided doses	Same as above	Less hypotension than phenytoin Bradycardia	Needs close drug-drug interaction monitoring due to strong CYP induction Max infusion rate: 150 mg/min Prodrug of phenytoin- takes ~15 min to convert to active drug Less thrombophlebitis than phenytoin
Valproic acid	LD: 20–40 mg/kg IVPB Maintenance: 10–15 mg/kg/day divided in 2–4 doses	Goal trough total level: 50–150 mcg/ml	Hyperammonemia Thrombocytopenia Hepatotoxicity	CYP enzyme inhibitor Frequency must be adjusted appropriately for formulation being utilized Free valproate levels are not routinely drawn in practice and must be sent out at most institutions
Levetiracetam	LD: 1–3 g IVPB or 60 mg/kg IVPB (max: 4.5 g) Maintenance: 750–1500 mg BID	Not routinely monitored	Somnolence Behavioral changes *may be increased in patients with history of psychiatric disorders	Must be renally dosed and supplemental doses provided with hemodialysis

| Phenobarbital | Loading dose: 15–20 mg/kg IVPB
Maintenance: 1–3 mg/kg/day in 1–3 divided doses | Goal trough levels: 15–40 mcg/ml *may need much higher serum concentrations if trying to achieve burst suppression | Hypotension
Sedation
Respiratory depression | Infusion rate: 50–100 mg/min
Needs close drug-drug interaction monitoring due to strong CYP induction
Do not load barbiturate naïve patients who are not intubated
Intermittent loads (for example to provide a load of 1200 mg give 300 mg by slow IVP every hour for 4 h) or slow infusion rate if patient experiences hypotension |
| Lacosamide | LD: 200–400 mg IVPB
Maintenance: 50–200 mg BID | Not routinely monitored | PR interval prolongation | Reduce dose in renal impairment and supplemental doses provided with hemodialysis
Monitor EKG for PR interval goal <200 |

Third Line Treatment

Drug	Dose	Target Drug Monitoring	Adverse Effects	Clinical Pearls
Midazolam	LD: 0.2 mg/kg IV bolus CI: 0.05–2 mg/kg/h For breakthrough SE: bolus 0.1–0.2 mg/kg AND increase CI by 0.05–0.1 mg/kg/h every 3–4 h	Titrate to EEG	Sedation Respiratory depression	Caution in patients with renal impairment due to accumulation of active metabolite Tachyphylaxis may occur after prolonged use
Propofol	LD: 1–2 mg/kg IV bolus (max: 200 mg)	Titrate to EEG	Hypotension Respiratory depression Sedation	Risk of PRIS is greatest in young patients, doses >67 mcg/kg/min and

Table 14.2 (cont.)

Third Line Treatment

Drug	Dose	Target Drug Monitoring	Adverse Effects	Clinical Pearls
	CI: 30–200 mcg/kg/min For breakthrough SE: increase CI by 5–10 mcg/kg/min every 5 min with or without a 1 mg/kg bolus		Propofol infusion syndrome (PRIS): severe metabolic acidosis, hyperkalemia, cardiac dysrhythmias, cardiovascular collapse, rhabdomyolysis	prolonged use >48 h. Monitor CK, lactate and TGs Dissolved in lipid emulsion delivering 1.1 kcal/ml
Pentobarbital	LD: 5–15 mg/kg IV bolus CI: 0.5–5 mg/kg/h For breakthrough SE: Bolus 5 mg/kg and increase CI by 0.5–1 mg/kg/h every 12 h	Titrate to EEG Therapeutic range: 10–20 mcg/ml (not routinely monitored)	Hypotension Sedation Respiratory depression Cardiac depression Paralytic ileus Loss of all neurologic function at high doses	Some patients may experience hemodynamic instability and will need vasopressor therapy Needs close drug–drug interaction monitoring due to strong CYP induction
Ketamine	LD: 1–2 mg/kg IV bolus CI: 0.6–10 mg/kg/h For breakthrough SE: Bolus 1–2 mg/kg and increase CI by 0.6 mg/kg/h	Titrate to EEG	Tachyarrhythmias Hypertension	Loading doses have been associated with transient hypotension

seizure suppression with either the same or alternative IV
anesthetics (i.e. ketamine or pentobarbital).
   c. Pharmacological options:
      a. Inhaled anesthetics (i.e. isoflurane)
      b. Addition of alternative AEDs (i.e. topiramate, carbamazepine,
         clobazam)
   d. Non-pharmacological options:
      a. Immune modulation: (IVIG, steroids, plasma exchange)
      b. Ketogenic diet
      c. IV magnesium
      d. Therapeutic hypothermia
      e. Electroconvulsive therapy
      f. Transmagnetic stimulation
      g. Neurosurgical evaluation

14.1.6.2   Treatment of Nonconvulsive Status Epilepticus

There is no universally accepted definition of nonconvulsive status
epilepticus (NCSE), and there is no consensus on how to treat it.
Once the diagnosis of NCSE is made there is often disagreement on
how aggressively it should be treated. This is particularly true when
patients with NCSE have only mild impairments in consciousness.
While human and animal data do suggest neuronal injury associated
with NCSE, aggressive treatments for nonconvulsive status epilepticus
are not benign. In clinical practice, the decision on how aggressively
to treat NCSE is based on the patient's mental status and clinical
course.[11] The treatment of NCSE follows the same algorithm as
convulsive status epilepticus with the caveat of risk-benefit analysis
regarding endotracheal intubation and use of IV anesthetics for
a patient with NCSE and retained consciousness. In all cases, it is
important to address the underlying cause of nonconvulsive status
epilepticus.

14.1.6.3   Treatment of Focal Status Epilepticus and Epilepsia Partialis Continua

Similar to the treatment of nonconvulsive status epilepticus there is a risk benefit analysis needed to decide how aggressive to be with treatment of focal status epilepticus and EPC that is based on the patient's mental status and clinical course. Overall, the treatment of focal status epilepticus is similar to the treatment algorithm for convulsive status epilepticus in regard to the first and second-line treatments. Whether to proceed with the more aggressive third-line treatments is based on clinical judgment made on a case-by-case basis.

14.1.7   STATUS EPILEPTICUS: PROGNOSIS

Three major factors determine the outcome in status epilepticus:[5,12]
1. The type of status epilepticus.
   a. Status epilepticus has an associated mortality of up to 30%.
   b. Refractory status epilepticus has an associated mortality of 16–39%.
   c. Super refractory status epilepticus has an associated mortality of 30–50%.
2. The duration of status epilepticus.
   a. Status epilepticus lasting longer than 1 h is associated with a 10-fold increase in mortality.
   b. Seizure control without need for deep suppression on EEG is associated with good functional recovery.
3. The etiology of status epilepticus.
   a. Status epilepticus associated with anoxia, intracranial hemorrhage, infections, tumors, and trauma are associated with higher mortality.

Other factors contributing to poor functional outcome following status epilepticus include: age over 60 years, female sex, treatment in smaller-sized hospitals, the presence of comorbidities (i.e. hypertension, diabetes, and prior stroke), and status epilepticus complications (i.e. respiratory failure and sepsis).

14.2 EEG Monitoring

EEG monitoring in the ICU is important for the diagnosis of subclinical and nonconvulsive seizures, particularly in patients with impaired mental status. In the medical ICU population, after excluding patients with clinical signs of seizures, approximately 8% of comatose patients are found to have electrographic seizures. This number is even larger within the neurological ICU where approximately 18% of patients with unexplained decreased consciousness have subclinical seizures on EEG.[13]

14.2.1 EEG INDICATIONS

Electrographic subclinical seizures and nonconvulsive status epilepticus are frequently seen following convulsive status epilepticus, particularly in patients with persistent poor mental status. Studies have reported subclinical seizures occurring in up to 48% and nonconvulsive status epilepticus in 14% of patients with apparent successful treatment of convulsive status epilepticus. In 2015, the Critical Care Continuous EEG Task Force of the American Clinical Neurophysiology Society released a consensus statement on the use of continuous EEG monitoring in critically ill adults and children to help guide the use of EEG in the ICU.[14]

Indications for continuous EEG in the ICU

1. Rule out subclinical or nonconvulsive seizures in patients with:
   a. Persistently impaired mental status following a convulsive seizure or convulsive status epilepticus.
   b. Ongoing frequently recurring subtle movements such as isolated eye movements that may or may not represent seizure activity.
   c. Impaired mental status in a patient with a history of epilepsy.
   d. Acute supratentorial brain injury with stupor or coma (i.e. traumatic brain injury, intracerebral hemorrhage, subarachnoid hemorrhage, acute ischemic stroke, encephalitis, and anoxic brain injury following cardiac arrest during and after therapeutic hypothermia).

e. Unexplained fluctuations in mental status without known acute brain injury.

2. Characterization of clinical paroxysmal events, such as tremors, rigidity, posturing, chewing, or autonomic spells of sudden hypertension, tachycardia, bradycardia, or apnea.

3. Evaluation of epileptiform activity seen on routine EEG.

4. Detection of cerebral ischemia (i.e. patients with subarachnoid hemorrhage who are at risk of delayed cerebral ischemia).

5. Requirement of pharmacologic paralysis with risk of seizures (i.e. refractory intracranial pressure or therapeutic hypothermia).

6. Titration of IV anesthetics for treatment of refractory status epilepticus.

14.2.2   DURATION OF EEG MONITORING

Continuous EEG monitoring should be initiated as soon as subclinical seizures are suspected, since prolonged nonconvulsive seizures and status epilepticus are associated with higher morbidity and mortality, and treatment is more likely to be effective earlier on in the course.

Consensus Recommendations for Duration of Continuous EEG Monitoring

1. Twenty-four hours of continuous EEG monitoring is recommended for most patients with concern for subclinical seizures.[14] This recommendation is based on prior studies showing that 88% of seizures are captured within the first 24 h of cEEG monitoring.

2. Special populations, such as patients with coma, periodic epileptiform discharges, or are pharmacologically sedated, may require longer monitoring, of up to 48 h or more.[14]

3. Continuous EEG monitoring should be continued while patients are on IV anesthetics for seizure suppression and cEEG should be continued for 24 h after IV anesthetics have been withdrawn to assure continued resolution of electrographic seizures.[14]

14.2.3 ICTAL-INTERICTAL CONTINUUM

The increased use of cEEG monitoring in the ICU has led to better detection of nonconvulsive status epilepticus; however, it has also led to increased detection of epileptiform patterns, referred to as the inter-ictal continuum, that are of unclear significance. These patterns are abnormal and can share features of ictal activity but do not meet criteria for definite electrographic seizures. It is unclear if these ictal-interictal patterns cause a similar degree of neuronal injury or poor neurologic outcome as are seen in electrographic seizures, and as such there is no clear consensus on how these patterns should be managed. Some experts advocate for empiric treatment trials with benzodiazepines or non-sedating AEDs in patients with high-risk ictal-interictal patterns (i.e. periodic discharges) and then monitoring for both clinical and electrographic improvement.[15] Unfortunately, this can be difficult to ascertain in critically ill patients with poor mental status and multiple medical comorbidities. Though there are no standardized guidelines for the management of ictal-interictal patterns, there is compelling evidence that some of these patterns are highly associated with seizures (Table 14.3) and may warrant extended monitoring.

14.3 Summary

Status epilepticus is a neurological emergency and is associated with high morbidity and mortality necessitating timely recognition and treatment. Prompt treatment with benzodiazepine followed by an anti-epileptic drug is crucial to reduce the risk of developing refractory status epilepticus. Continuous EEG monitoring is essential for both recognizing nonconvulsive status epilepticus and titrating IV anesthetics in the treatment of refractory status epilepticus. Early treatment and stabilization along with simultaneous diagnostic evaluation are imperative for successful resolution of status epilepticus.

Table 14.3 Ictal-interictal patterns: etiology and association with seizures

Pattern	Etiology	Association with Seizures
Lateralized Periodic Discharges (LPDs)	Typically found in association with acute or chronic structural brain abnormality Examples: stroke, tumors, encephalitis, traumatic brain injury, and intracerebral hemorrhage	High association with seizures: 40–95%
Bilateral Independent Periodic Discharges (BIPDs)	Typically found in acute or subacute bi-hemispheric brain injury Examples: CNS infection, anoxic injury, tumors, stroke, and metabolic disturbances	High association with seizures: 43–78%
Generalized Periodic Discharges (GPDs)	Typically associated with severe encephalopathy or coma and tends to reflect diffuse global brain dysfunction Examples: toxic-metabolic disturbances, sepsis, acute brain injury, hypoxic injury, Creutzfeldt Jacob Disease	Association with seizures: 20–26%
Triphasic Waves (TW)	TW are a subset of GPDs that are typically found in association with metabolic disturbance Examples: hepatic encephalopathy, hyponatremia, hypothyroid states, sepsis, lithium toxicity, cefepime toxicity, hypertensive encephalopathy	Association with seizures: similar to that of other PDs

Lateralized Rhythmic Delta Activity (LRDA)	Typically associated with acute or remote focal CNS lesions Examples: frequently seen in ICH and SAH	High association with seizures: ~53%
Generalized Rhythmic Delta Activity (GRDA)	Typically associated with various degrees of encephalopathy, but also can be seen in association with deep midline structural lesions and increased intracranial pressure in the appropriate clinical context	Low association with seizures
Stimulus-Induced Rhythmic Periodic or Ictal Discharges (SIRPIDs)	Typically seen in acute brain injury Examples: stroke, ICH, SAH, TBI, anoxic injury, neurodegenerative disorders, metabolic disturbances	No clear consensus

References

1. Brophy GM, et al. Guidelines for the evaluation and management of status epilepticus. Neurocrit Care. 2012;17(1):3–23.

2. Wasterlain CG, Chen JW. Mechanistic and pharmacologic aspects of status epilepticus and its treatment with new antiepileptic drugs. Epilepsia. 2008;49(Suppl 9):63–73.

3. Meldrum BS, Brierley JB. Prolonged epileptic seizures in primates: ischemic cell change and its relation to ictal physiological events. Arch Neurol. 1973;28(1):10–17.

4. Sánchez S, Rincon F. Status epilepticus: epidemiology and public health needs. J Clin Med. August 16, 2016;5(8):71. doi:10.3390/jcm5080071.

5. Nelson SE, Varelas PN. Status epilepticus, refractory status epilepticus, and super-refractory status epilepticus. Continuum (Minneap Minn). 2018;24(6):1683–707.

6. Trinka E, et al. A definition and classification of status epilepticus – Report of the ILAE Task Force on Classification of Status Epilepticus. Epilepsia. 2015;56(10):1515–23.

7. Treiman DM. A comparison of four treatments for generalized convulsive status epilepticus. N Engl J Med. 1998;339(12):792–98.

8. Silbergleit R, et al. RAMPART (Rapid Anticonvulsant Medication Prior to Arrival Trial): a double-blind randomized clinical trial of the efficacy of intramuscular midazolam versus intravenous lorazepam in the prehospital treatment of status epilepticus by paramedics. Epilepsia. 2011;52(Suppl 8):45–47.

9. Glauser T. Evidence based guideline: treatment of convulsive status epilepticus in children and adults. Epilepsy Currents. 2016;16:48–61.

10. Kapur J, et al. Randomized trial of three anticonvulsant medications for status epilepticus. N Engl J Med. 2019;381(22):2103–13.

11. VanHaerents S, Gerard EE. Epilepsy emergencies: status epilepticus, acute repetitive seizures, and autoimmune encephalitis. Continuum (Minneap Minn). 2019;25 (2):454–76.

12. DeLorenzo RJ, et al. A prospective, population-based epidemiologic study of status epilepticus in Richmond, Virginia. Neurology. 1996;46(4):1029–35.

13. Claassen J, et al. Detection of electrographic seizures with continuous EEG monitoring in critically ill patients. Neurology. 2004;62(10):1743–48.

14. Herman S, Abend N, Bleck T. Consensus statement on continuous EEG in critically ill adults and children. J Clin Neurophysiol. 2015;32:87–95.

15. Cormier J, Maciel CB, Gilmore EJ. Ictal-interictal continuum: when to worry about the continuous electroencephalography pattern. Semin Respir Crit Care Med. 2017;38 (6):793–806.

15

Evaluation of the Comatose Patient and Overview of the Brain Death Examination

Sherri A Braksick and Alejandro A Rabinstein

Abstract

An acutely comatose patient is a medical emergency that requires rapid evaluation and initiation of management of the underlying cause, whether it is due to a primary neurologic insult or secondary to a serious medical condition. Often, the most important details are obtained from a direct witness to the event that can provide information about the events leading up to the presentation and the patient's medical history and medication usage. The physical examination provides clues to help localize the region of the central nervous system affected, helping to narrow the differential diagnosis. Diagnostic testing is tailored to the medical history and examination. Regardless of the ultimate cause, prompt initiation of treatment is imperative to provide the patient the best opportunity to recover. The diagnosis of brain death is a clinical diagnosis, and should be completed in a structured, stepwise manner. Ancillary testing should only be obtained if the clinical examination is unable to be fully completed.

15.1 Introduction

An acutely comatose patient is alarming to both neurologists and non-neurologists. Unresponsiveness can occur due to many different reasons, and be due to primary neurologic injury or occur as a manifestation of severe systemic illnesses. Discriminating between the broad differential diagnoses requires a thoughtful, stepwise process that is tailored to each patient based on known medical comorbidities, time course of events and the patient's recent medical history.

15.2 Evaluation of a Comatose Patient

15.2.1 OBTAINING THE HISTORY

Correctly obtaining from a witness the sequence of events leading up to the patient's comatose state is imperative. Often, at the time of the initial assessment, these witnesses may still be en route to the hospital, but this step cannot be overlooked and contacting them by phone whenever possible will help provide the most appropriate care to the patient.

In order to fully understand the situation, the rapidity of symptom onset, any preceding symptoms, recent illnesses, current medications, recently increased or discontinued medications, illicit substance use (including alcohol and illegal drugs), recent trauma, risks for suicidality and known existing medical problems all need to be reviewed. When done correctly, this information can often help to substantially narrow the differential diagnosis.[1]

Key historical components in an acutely comatose or unresponsive patient are listed in Table 15.1.

15.2.2 IDENTIFYING CONFOUNDERS TO THE EXAMINATION

Patients who are found unresponsive are often urgently intubated for airway protection, prior to transport to the hospital or shortly after arrival to the emergency room. Medications used for intubation

Table 15.1 Important historical details in acute unresponsiveness

Details of current episode

Onset – progressive vs. sudden	Exact sequence of events from a first-person witness – best obtained in a stepwise manner (e.g. Then what happened?)	Location/setting where unresponsiveness occurred (e.g. work, home, hospital, etc.)
Trauma	Prodromal symptoms – headache, fever, weakness, abnormal movements	Time the patient was "last known well"
Alcohol use	Medications taken (prescription and over-the-counter)	Illicit substances taken

Medical history

Medical history – concise but thorough (stroke risk factors, history of neurologic disease, kidney/liver disease, etc.)	Recent illnesses	Prescribed medication list
Potential for medication errors	Over-the-counter medications	Drug abuse history
Alcohol use history	Recent medication changes (additions or deletions)	Recent life events (including good and bad stressors)
Recent psychiatric history (depression, recent mood changes, hallucinations)	Risk factors for drug/medication withdrawal (financial issues, etc.)	

substantially confound and essentially eliminate the ability to obtain a neurologic examination, with the exception of pupillary responses, which should be present even shortly after the use of a paralytic. When evaluating a poorly responsive patient, it is important to note what medications are currently being infused, and also to review with the nurse the last doses of sedating medications (e.g. opioids, benzodiazepines) given to the patient.

Other important confounders to the examination include untreated hypothermia or severe fever, both of which can result in decreased responsiveness. A hypotensive patient can also be poorly responsive due to impaired cerebral perfusion. It is fairly easy to determine if a patient has fluctuating responsiveness due to impaired perfusion by comparing examinations with the head of the bed at 30–45° and then with the patient supine or in Trendelenburg position (once increased intracranial pressure is excluded).

15.2.3   COMMON COMA SCALES

There are two major scores utilized by neurologists to characterize a patient's responsiveness, the Glasgow Coma Scale (GCS)[2] and the Full Outline of UnResponsiveness (FOUR Score).[3] Coma scales provide a method to communicate a patient's condition to other providers and also allow for a standardized assessment of clinical change over time. Both scores can be completed efficiently at the bedside within 1–2 min and have been found to be valid and reliable. The presence of confounders to these assessments (e.g. ongoing sedation or opioid infusions, hypothermia, etc.) should be noted and recorded when the examination is documented to provide a full clinical illustration of the patient's condition.

15.2.3.1   Glasgow Coma Scale

The GCS was developed in 1974 (originally designed for evaluation in the field of patients with head trauma) and over the subsequent decades has become a common tool used to describe the examination in poorly responsive patients. This score includes three separate components: eye response, verbal response, and motor response, with a minimum total score of three and maximum of 15. (Table 15.2) The

Table 15.2 Glasgow coma scale

Score		Glasgow Coma Scale	
	Eye	Verbal	Motor
0	NA	NA	NA
1	No eye opening	No verbal response	No motor response
2	Eyes open to pain	Incomprehensible sounds	Extensor response to pain
3	Eyes open to voice	Inappropriate words	Flexion response to pain
4	Eyes spontaneously open	Confused	Withdrawal from pain
5	NA	Oriented	Localizing to pain
6	NA	NA	Follows commands

GCS continues to be a popular tool to facilitate communication between providers and has also been included in some prognostic scales. Treatment decisions based on the sum score (e.g. intubate for GCS <8) have been proposed, though this may oversimplify decisions in patients with pre-existing disability or speech disorders where a baseline GCS may not be normal.

15.2.3.2 Full Outline of UnResponsiveness (FOUR) Score

The FOUR Score is a newer coma scale with a maximum score of 16 and minimum of zero. This scale utilizes four components, each with four possible points. (Table 15.3) This scale records evaluation of eye-opening and motor response, similar to the GCS, but also includes brain stem reflexes and respiratory pattern, allowing the physician to localize the disorder in addition to grading the degree of abnormality on the examination. The FOUR score does not include a verbal component, and consequently, it does not lose discriminative ability in intubated patients, unlike the GCS.

Table 15.3 The full outline of unresponsiveness (FOUR Score)

FOUR Score			
Eye	Motor	Brain stem	Respiratory
0 No eye opening	No motor response or generalized myoclonus	Absent pupil, corneal and cough reflexes	Does not breathe above the set ventilator rate
1 Eyes open to pain	Extension response to pain	Pupil and corneal responses absent	Intubated, breathing above the ventilator rate
2 Eyes open to voice	Flexion response to pain	Pupil or corneal response absent	Irregular breathing
3 Eyes open, not tracking	Localizes to pain	One pupil wide and fixed	Cheyne-Stokes respiratory pattern
4 Eyes open, tracking	Follows commands	Pupil and corneal responses present	Regular breathing pattern

15.2.4   OTHER EXAMINATION FINDINGS AND LESION LOCALIZATION

15.2.4.1   Motor Examination

Simple observation can be extremely informative when determining the level of consciousness of a patient, and asymmetry of motor movements can point to a focal lesion even before formal testing is initiated.

Abnormal movements are often best seen during a short period of observation upon entrance to the patient's room. Diffuse myoclonus is frequently due to toxic or metabolic derangements, such as CO_2 narcosis, opioid use or renal impairment. Asterixis (negative myoclonus) is best noted after raising the patient's arm. It is more common in liver failure but can also be seen with other toxic and metabolic encephalopathies. The lack of rhythmicity of myoclonus is usually sufficient to differentiate it from seizures. Yet, post-anoxic myoclonus can be associated with epileptic changes on EEG.

Evaluation of muscle tone is important. Comatose patients are often hypotonic, but any hypertonicity is more informative. Hypertonicity may be due to spasticity or rigidity. Asymmetric spasticity often indicates an upper motor neuron lesion of the contralateral side of the brain that can be acute, subacute, or chronic. Asymmetric rigidity may be seen in movement disorders that result in Parkinsonism or with lesions to the basal ganglia and its circuits. Presence of greater rigidity in the legs than in the arms, particularly when accompanied by lower extremity clonus, should prompt consideration of serotonin syndrome. Generalized rigidity may represent neuroleptic malignant syndrome in the proper clinical context, and can also be seen in dopamine-withdrawal states or in some autoimmune conditions.

Motor responses should be evaluated with central and peripheral painful stimulation. Central stimulation can be produced by pressing on the temporomandibular joints or the supraorbital notches. Peripheral stimulation is typically generated by applying pressure to nailbeds. All extremities should be individually tested. Best responses of each extremity should be documented and any asymmetry should be highlighted.

Posturing is a concerning finding, and should raise suspicion for a structural brain injury. Extensor posturing (decerebrate) can occur as a consequence of a brain stem injury distal to the red nucleus in the midbrain and above the vestibular nucleus in the lower pons. Flexor (decorticate) posturing often indicates a lesion in the upper brain stem – above the red nucleus. In focal cortical lesions, asymmetry of posturing can also occur.

15.2.4.2   Nuchal Rigidity

All comatose patients should be assessed for nuchal rigidity, a finding that may suggest meningeal irritation, principally from infection. Meningeal signs have overall poor sensitivity,[4] but, when present, should strongly encourage evaluation for CNS infection, as the consequences of a missed diagnosis can be catastrophic.

15.2.4.3 Pupillary and Eye Examination

Many clues to the cause and severity of CNS pathology can sometimes be found with a simple examination of a patient's eyes. The presence of a gaze deviation indicates damage to the ipsilateral frontal eye field, as in stroke or tumor, or inappropriate activation of the contralateral frontal eye field, which can be seen in ongoing seizure. A post-ictal patient may present with gaze deviation toward the side opposite the seizure focus and, if a Todd's paralysis is present, may be mistaken for a stroke, emphasizing the need for an accurate history of all events preceding the patient's presentation.

Ocular bobbing (vertical, involuntary movements) may indicate brain stem disease, possibly of the pons, but this is difficult to precisely localize. The presence of a skew deviation (i.e. vertical misalignment) should likewise cause concern for brain stem pathology. A dysconjugate gaze (i.e. horizontal misalignment) can be seen in deep coma states or be secondary to sedation and often has no localizing value, though they can occasionally signal brain stem disease.

Subtle nystagmoid eye movements may be the only manifestation in some patients with status epilepticus. Thus, detailed examination of the eyes should be prolonged for a few minutes, especially when non-convulsive seizures are considered possible.

The pupillary examination can point to emergent pathology that requires rapid management. The so-called blown pupil, a unilateral, large, and unreactive pupil in an acutely comatose patient is suggestive of uncal herniation, and should prompt initiation of treatment for increased intracranial pressure. However, direct injury to a cranial nerve or ocular trauma can also cause a large, unreactive pupil in the absence of herniation. In large supratentorial lesions, patients may develop bilateral fixed and unreactive pupils due to compression of the midbrain and exiting third cranial nerves bilaterally. Pontine injuries can lead to very small, but persistently reactive, pupils, similar to those seen in patients who have received opioid medications.

15.2.4.4 Systemic Examination

In addition to a thorough neurologic examination, other data, such as vital signs and the systemic examination, may suggest the underlying cause of the patient's unresponsive state.

The presence of a hypersympathetic state (fever, mydriasis, diaphoresis, tachycardia, etc.) may be indicative of ingestion of sympathomimetics, withdrawal from a CNS depressant medication, serotonin syndrome, or neuroleptic malignant syndrome.

The presence of fever should prompt concern for infection of the CNS or systemically, and in the setting of unresponsiveness, may warrant evaluation of cerebrospinal fluid.

A full skin assessment should be performed to evaluate for rashes, such as seen with Neisseria meningitides infection. Other stigmata of potential autoimmunity (e.g. livedo reticularis, malar rash) should be noted as well. Completion of a full skin assessment will also allow the examiner to assess for evidence of trauma, including Battle's sign behind an ear that is seen in basilar skull fractures, or bruising that would otherwise be hidden by a hospital gown or clothing.

Other findings that should actively be sought in an unresponsive patient include evidence of puncture marks from drug use, a cardiac murmur if there is concern for sepsis and endocarditis, a tongue bite that may suggest seizure and any unusual odors on the patient's clothing or breath that may suggest a toxic ingestion or a metabolic disorder.

15.3 Differential Diagnosis in Coma

The differential diagnosis of an acutely unresponsive patient is extensive, but it often can be narrowed after a detailed physical examination and understanding of the patient's presenting history and known medical problems. Unfortunately, a neurologist is often asked to evaluate the patient shortly after receiving sedating medications for one of several reasons, which forces the physician to maintain a broad differential until information becomes clearer.

Localizing findings on an examination, such as an asymmetric motor exam (e.g. in the degree of movement or in tone), pupillary asymmetry or the presence of a gaze deviation, are suggestive of a structural lesion, which can help guide initial diagnostic steps. In the proper clinical context, the classic "locked-in" syndrome should be excluded by asking the patient to look up and down, to ensure alertness is not overlooked in patients who otherwise appear comatose. Locked-in patients will often have pinpoint pupils with extensor posturing of the upper extremities to pain, and will have their eyes closed at rest.

Focal findings can occasionally be explained by less concerning reasons, such as a patient presenting with acute sepsis and reemergence of a prior neurologic deficit from multiple sclerosis or stroke. These patients may have had a previous neurologic deficit that improved with time, but in the setting of acute decompensation (often infection), these prior deficits may re-emerge, only to recover again when the primary medical issue is managed.[5]

Often, unresponsive patients have intact brain stem reflexes and an otherwise symmetric, though poor, neurologic examination. These patients can present a diagnostic challenge, as this implies a non-focal, bihemispheric dysfunction, frequently due to toxic/metabolic or systemic disorders. Rarely, a primary neurologic disorder can present in this manner, such as nonconvulsive status epilepticus.

A comprehensive list of differential diagnoses is listed in Table 15.4, organized by lesion localization.

15.4 Diagnostic Testing

The choice of diagnostic testing in an acutely comatose patient will be somewhat variable and dependent on the history and examination. Often,

Table 15.4 Differential diagnosis in acute coma

Intact brain stem and symmetric motor responses	Abnormal brain stem examination
Toxic/Metabolic Causes	Acute basilar artery occlusion (ischemic stroke) – evaluate for locked-in state
Severe sepsis	Uncal or downward herniation (due to hemispheric stroke, tumor, diffuse cerebral edema, etc.)
Hypoperfusion state (shock)	Intrinsic brain stem tumor or hemorrhage
Hypercapnia/Hypoxia	
Carbon Monoxide Poisoning	
Medication overdose	**Intact brain stem with asymmetric motor responses**
Unknown toxidrome	Large hemispheric stroke
Illicit drug use/overdose (including synthetic marijuana and opioid products)	Bilateral hemispheric strokes
Alcohol ingestion (ethanol or atypical alcohols; including in-hospital ingestion of hand sanitizer)	Intracerebral hemorrhage
Persistent medication effect	Subdural/epidural hemorrhage
Impaired medication clearance: liver/renal impairment	Aneurysmal subarachnoid hemorrhage (often non-focal presentation)
Acute liver failure and hyperammonemia	Intracranial abscess
Hyperammonemia in the absence of liver failure	Hemispheric tumor with mass effect
Hyper/hypoglycemia	Recrudescence of prior deficits (from stroke or multiple sclerosis) in the setting of a systemic infection
Hyper/hyponatremia	Cerebral air or fat embolism
Multiple, mild electrolyte abnormalities	Tumefactive multiple sclerosis
Serotonin Syndrome	Acute disseminated encephalomyelitis (ADEM)

Table 15.4 (cont.)

Intact brain stem and symmetric motor responses	Abnormal brain stem examination
Neuroleptic malignant syndrome/ dopamine withdrawal, malignant catatonia	
Endocrine abnormalities (Myxedema coma, adrenal insufficiency)	
Pituitary apoplexy and secondary adrenal insufficiency	
Nonconvulsive Status Epilepticus	
Posterior Reversible Encephalopathy Syndrome	
Infectious meningitis/encephalitis	
Non-infectious (autoimmune) encephalitis	
Venous sinus thrombosis	
Aneurysmal subarachnoid hemorrhage	
Bilateral thalamic strokes	
Acute or progressive hydrocephalus	

with a clear understanding of the patient's presentation and clinical findings, the evaluation can be approached in a stepwise manner, looking for the most likely and emergent cause initially, and subsequently casting a wider net if an etiology is not initially discovered. Common tests in an unresponsive patient are listed in Table 15.5.

15.4.1 RADIOGRAPHIC EVALUATION

Acutely comatose patients should undergo head imaging to ensure there are no underlying structural causes, such as hemorrhage, tumor, or occult stroke. A non-contrast computed tomography (CT) scan of the head is the first study that should be completed, and is often obtained even prior to a neurologic consultation. This study is rapidly available and will readily identify hemorrhage, most tumors if there is associated edema, and subacute or chronic ischemic strokes. Acute strokes and small lesions may not be visible on CT scan, and if clinical suspicion is high, these should continue to be considered and further evaluated or empirically treated.

Advanced imaging with magnetic resonance (MRI) should be considered to further evaluate an abnormality seen on an initial CT scan or if suspicion remains high for a focal lesion not previously visualized. Based on the patient's comorbidity (e.g. known systemic cancer, renal function), physicians will need to determine if contrast is warranted (e.g. when looking for tumors or suspected meningitis) and safe to administer. MRI may not be rapidly available, and becomes more cumbersome to arrange in intubated patients.

In patients with focal neurologic findings, such as an asymmetric motor examination or abnormalities of brain stem reflexes, the possibility of acute stroke needs to be considered. In these situations where there is potential for a large vessel occlusion (e.g. carotid, middle cerebral, basilar), a CT angiogram should be done to ensure patency of vessels or to confirm the suspected occlusion, which can facilitate triage and potential endovascular therapy. It is important to realize that acute strokes do not often result in coma or poor responsiveness, though this may occur with lesions affecting substantial portions of a cerebral hemisphere, bilateral hemispheres, the brain stem, or thalamus.

15.4.2 LABORATORY EVALUATION

Initial laboratory for comatose patients should include a complete blood count, with special attention to leukocytes, as well as a full metabolic panel, evaluating for electrolyte abnormalities, and liver or renal impairment. Depending on patient comorbidity, additional evaluation of coagulation parameters (prothrombin time, activated partial thromboplastin time and international normalized ratio – INR), ammonia and endocrine studies (thyroid function and rarely, cortisol) should be considered as well.

If the presenting syndrome is unclear or concerning for infection – particularly with the presence of fever or hypothermia – blood cultures should be obtained prior to initiation of any antimicrobials, if this will not delay treatment.

Urine studies, including a basic urinalysis, gram stain and toxicology screen can help identify other causes of unresponsiveness. It is important to note that urine drug screens will often fail to identify some illicit substances, including – but not limited to – synthetic opioids, and specific evaluation for particular substances may need to be requested separately. Additionally, some toxic substances or poisons are best evaluated with serum studies, and the preferred method for specific compounds should be reviewed by the ordering physician, or in consultation with the local poison control center if suspicion is high.

If the cause of a patient's acute coma/unresponsiveness remains elusive beyond initial imaging and basic serological studies, physicians should consider performing a lumbar puncture to evaluate for acute infection, particularly if the patient is febrile or has leukocytosis. When a lumbar puncture is being completed for a concern of infection, blood cultures should also be obtained and empiric coverage should be initiated, even before the lumbar puncture is completed. (Initiation of antibiotics should not obviate the emergent need for cerebrospinal fluid sampling, which should be obtained as soon as it is safe and feasible, as delays in fluid collection will decrease the likelihood of identifying the causative infectious agent.) Basic studies on the cerebrospinal fluid should include cell count with differential, protein, glucose, bacterial gram stain and culture, herpes simplex PCRs and cytology. Additional studies are

Table 15.5 Diagnostic testing in an unresponsive patient

First-line tests (done in nearly all patients)	Other considerations (dependent on the patient's exam/history)
Point of care glucose	Vascular imaging of the brain (CT angiogram)
Complete blood count	Lumbar puncture to evaluate for infection
Comprehensive metabolic panel	Serological/urine studies for specific toxins/ suspected ingestions
Serum ammonia	Electroencephalogram
Thyroid function studies	Magnetic Resonance Imaging (MRI) head
Arterial blood gas	Brain imaging (CT or MRI) with contrast
Serum lactic acid	Autoimmune evaluation (anti-nuclear antibody, antibodies to extractable nuclear antigens, etc.)
Urine drug screen	Paraneoplastic antibodies – considered after other more acute studies have been completed
Urinalysis with gram stain	
Blood cultures	
Tracheal secretion cultures (if present)	
Portable chest X-ray	
Non-contrast CT scan of the head	

dependent on the clinical situation and patient comorbidity. An overview of diagnostic testing is listed in Table 15.5.

15.4.3 ELECTROENCEPHALOGRAM

In some patients, the need for an electroencephalogram (EEG) is clear – the patient had a witnessed event concerning for seizure, and has since been unresponsive. Other patients have a history of epilepsy and were "found down," a common scenario that often warrants a short-term EEG, at a minimum. EEG monitoring should be pursued in patients who present with one or more witnessed seizures and do not begin to wake up promptly (e.g. within 1 h) of their last clinical event, to ensure there are not ongoing non-convulsive seizures. The indication for EEG monitoring is less robust in unresponsive patients with a non-focal neurologic examination and no clear risk factors for seizures, but EEG should be considered when the cause of the coma remains unclear.

A fairly recent study found non-convulsive seizures in 29% of patients who presented with altered mental status. However, if patients did not have evidence of epileptiform abnormality within the first 4 h after the EEG was initiated, no subsequent seizures were found on prolonged monitoring.[6] This implies that in cases where continuous EEG is utilized, if no clear epileptiform abnormalities are seen in the first several hours of recording, the likelihood of subsequent seizures (in the absence of additional risk factors for their development) is negligible.

15.5 Management of the Comatose Patient

The management of a comatose patient is primarily dependent on the underlying cause, though adequate supportive care is also essential. Patients presenting with acute coma to the Emergency Department should receive thiamine before they receive any glucose.

Primary neurologic disorders causing coma or poor responsiveness (e.g. stroke, status epilepticus) are discussed elsewhere in this book. Patients with medical conditions that result in coma, such as severe sepsis and acute liver or renal failure, require urgent management of the underlying condition and time to allow the patient to recover. In patients with severe abnormalities of liver and kidney function, the effects of sedating medications should be expected to persist for a prolonged period of time. Additionally, hyperammonemia requires aggressive treatment, as this condition can result in cerebral edema that requires ongoing monitoring, and potentially osmotherapy while the primary cause of liver impairment is treated.

In toxidromes, physicians must determine if enteric administration of activated charcoal or other treatments to prevent absorption are indicated. Specific antidotes should be sought and administered in the proper clinical context. All toxidromes and medication overdoses should be discussed with the local toxicologist and poison control center to help guide management.

15.5.1 MANAGING ELEVATED INTRACRANIAL PRESSURE

Increased intracranial pressure may be the cause of coma or poor responsiveness, either due to a structural abnormality due to acute CSF outflow obstruction, or as a consequence of another disorder (e.g. hydrocephalus secondary to impaired arachnoid granulation function or diffuse cerebral edema secondary to acute liver failure). Specific management of elevated ICP is discussed elsewhere in this text, and we refer the reader to the dedicated chapter on this topic.

15.5.2 OTHER CONSIDERATIONS

Comatose patients will clearly have impaired mobility and will require intensive care for management of all of their needs. Excellent nursing care, with frequent repositioning to prevent pressure ulcerations, and hygiene to prevent skin breakdown are paramount. Good respiratory hygiene and repositioning the resting position of the endotracheal tube by respiratory therapy can prevent pressure ulcers of the mouth as well.

The intensive care team must ensure adequate nutrition is provided, stress ulcer prophylaxis is administered to intubated patients, and deep vein thrombosis prevention techniques using sequential compression devices and/or prophylactic doses of heparin or enoxaparin are used. A scheduled bowel regimen may also be necessary to prevent the development of ileus.

15.6 The Brain Death Examination

The concept of brain death has been discussed in the literature for many years, and in the United States was formally defined in 1981 as an irreversible cessation of entire brain function, including the brain stem.[7] Subsequently, the American Academy of Neurology (AAN) developed a practice parameter to determine brain death in adults,[8] and a separate pediatric guideline was developed and endorsed by multiple medical societies.[9] Children under 18 years of age require two separate examinations (the duration between examinations differs based on the patient's age).

Each individual state and hospital have specified requirements for brain death determination, often taken from, or at least influenced by, the formal guidelines. Physicians should be familiar with their specific state and institutional policies, as some will require multiple examinations for both pediatric and adult patients, and examination recommendations may differ from the evidence-based guidelines. This section will focus on the process of brain death determination in an adult, based on the current AAN practice parameter.

It is the responsibility of the physician to determine that performing a formal brain death examination is appropriate for each patient. This examination should not be considered an emergent procedure, but rather must be treated with utmost respect to protect the integrity of the death declaration. Organ procurement organizations (OPOs) are often aware of potential organ donors prior to brain death declaration, however, these organizations should have no role in the diagnosis of death, including the timing of the examination, and should only be formally involved and approach families regarding the potential for donation after death declaration. Physicians caring for a patient should not be involved in organ donation decisions or discuss organ donation with families.

15.6.1 PREREQUISITES PRIOR TO THE EXAMINATION

Arguably the most important consideration in brain death determination is ensuring that a patient has suffered an irreversible brain injury, and is able to undergo the examination in the absence of confounders, which should be considered the first step of the formal examination. Hospitalized, intubated patients have typically during the hospitalization been exposed to sedating medications at some point of their admission. The circumstances surrounding the patient's brain injury may also be secondary to confounding medications (opioid-induced anoxic brain injury, for example). In addition to medication effects, ongoing metabolic derangements should be identified and corrected. Irreversibility is determined by imaging findings and physician understanding of the physiologic implications of such.

The AAN guideline has outlined specific confounders which may affect the integrity of the brain death examination, and these should be reviewed in a checklist manner by the physician and team performing the examination.

All of the following *must be true* prior to proceeding with the physical examination:

- Coma, irreversible and cause known
- Neuroimaging explains coma
- Sedative drug effect absent (obtain a toxicology screen if indicated)
- No residual effect of paralytic drug (check train-of-four if indicated)
- Absence of severe acid-base, electrolyte or endocrine abnormality
- Normal or near-normal temperature (core temperature ≥36 °C)
- Systolic blood pressure ≥100 mmHg
- No spontaneous respirations

15.6.2 THE EXAMINATION

Once irreversibility has been determined and confounders have been excluded, the formal brain death examination can proceed. This examination should be completed in a stepwise manner without omissions (with few exceptions, discussed in Section 15.6.4) and should include an evaluation for evidence of brain stem and cortical response to various stimuli.

- ○ Pupils non-reactive to bright light (pupils will typically be 5–7 mm in size)
- ○ Corneal response absent bilaterally
- ○ Oculocephalic response is absent (eyes remain immobile with head turn; defer in the presence of cervical spine injury)
- ○ Oculovestibular (caloric) response absent bilaterally (using 50 mL of ice water in each ear sequentially)
- ○ No facial movement to central noxious stimulus (supraorbital nerve and/or temporomandibular joint compression)
- ○ Absent gag reflex
- ○ Cough reflex is absent to deep endotracheal suctioning reaching the carina (perform at least 2 passes)
- ○ No motor response to peripheral noxious stimulus (perform painful stimulus in all four limbs). Spinally mediated reflexes (e.g. triple flexion) are permitted and can be recognized by their invariability.

15.6.3   APNEA TESTING

If no evidence of response is found on the above physical examination, the final portion of the brain death examination is performance of an apnea test. Apnea testing can be completed safely in the great majority of patients if proper procedures are strictly followed. Rarely, patients with very severe lung injury or cardiac disease/arrhythmias may not be stable enough to tolerate this examination; in such cases, an ancillary test is necessary to complement the clinical examination in the assessment of brain death. Proper apnea testing must proceed along the following steps:

- Ensure the patient is hemodynamically stable with a blood pressure $\geq$100 mmHg systolic. Vasopressors can be used and titrated to maintain this goal.
- Adjust the ventilator to achieve normocapnia ($PaCO_2$ between 35 and 45 mmHg) and confirm it has been achieved prior to apnea testing.
- Pre-oxygenate the patient with 100% FIO_2 for approximately 10 min, and confirm $PaO_2 \geq 200$ mmHg prior to testing.
- Ensure oxygenation can be maintained with a PEEP of 5 cm H_2O.
- Bare the patient's chest and abdomen to allow for observation of respiratory effort.
- Disconnect the ventilator and provide oxygen via an insufflation catheter at the level of the carina set to 6 L/min, or use a T-piece catheter and CPAP valve set to 10–20 cm H_2O. Do not titrate oxygen delivery rates during the apnea test.
- Monitor the patient by direct observation for 8–10 min, looking carefully for evidence of respiratory effort.
- If no respirations are seen, measure arterial blood gases at 8–10 min and reconnect the patient to the ventilator.
- If the $PaCO_2$ increases by at least 20 mmHg from the baseline value or is $\geq$60 mmHg, the patient is declared brain dead, and the time of death is the time the blood for $PaCO_2$ measurement was collected.

Rarely patients will not tolerate apnea testing due to hemodynamic instability or rapid desaturation. In such cases, the physician should consider aborting the test and repeating the apnea test at a later time or proceeding with an ancillary test.

15.6.4   ROLE OF ANCILLARY TESTS

Ancillary testing is recommended in situations where clinical factors prevent a full physical examination (extensive facial fractures, cervical spine injury, etc.) or if hemodynamic instability or very severe lung injury prevents a complete apnea test. Ancillary testing should not be considered a substitute for the clinical examination, which is the gold standard for the diagnosis of brain death.

15.6.4.1 Acceptable Ancillary Tests

Multiple electrical or cerebral blood flow tests have been used and are considered acceptable ancillary tests in brain death. These include a nuclear medicine scan, cerebral angiography, electroencephalography (EEG), CT angiogram, MRI/MRA, and transcranial Doppler studies. All of these tests have standard methods outlined in the brain death guideline that must be met to be considered acceptable for use in helping to determine brain death.

In situations where an ancillary test is used in the determination of brain death (which should only be completed following an attempted clinical brain death examination), the time of death is the time of the test's formal report of complete absence of cerebral blood flow or electrical activity.

15.7 Conclusions

The evaluation of an acutely comatose patient requires the physician to be efficient and thorough. The most important component of the evaluation is an accurate history of the events leading up to presentation, knowledge of the patient's current medications, recent medication changes and a clear understanding of the patient's medical history. A complete physical exam can assist in neurologic localization and identify systemic findings that may further narrow the differential diagnosis. A tailored evaluation with laboratory and radiographic studies often leads to the underlying cause to further guide ongoing management.

Brain death determination is a clinical diagnosis, and ancillary testing should only be considered when patient factors (e.g. extensive facial trauma, severe ARDS) prevent a full bedside examination.

References

1. Rabinstein AA. Coma and brain death. Continuum. 2018;24(6):1708-31.

2. Teasdale G, Jennett B. Assessment of coma and impaired consciousness: a practical scale. Lancet. 1974;2(7872):81-84.

3. Wijdicks EF, et al. Validation of a new coma scale: the FOUR score. Ann Neurol. 2005;58 (4):585-93.

4. Thomas KE, et al. The diagnostic accuracy of Kernig's sign, Brudzinski's sign, and nuchal rigidity in adults with suspected meningitis. Clin Infect Dis. 2002;35(1):46-52.

5. Berkovich RR. Acute multiple sclerosis relapse. Continuum (Minneap Minn). 2016;22 (3):799 814.

6. Shafi MM, et al. Absence of early epileptiform abnormalities predicts lack of seizures on continuous EEG. Neurology. 2012;79(17):1796-801.

7. Guidelines for the determination of death. Report of the medical consultants on the diagnosis of death to the President's Commission for the Study of Ethical Problems in Medicine and Biomedical and Behavioral Research. JAMA. 1981;246(19):2184-86.

8. Wijdicks EF, et al. Evidence-based guideline update: determining brain death in adults: report of the Quality Standards Subcommittee of the American Academy of Neurology. Neurology. 2010;74(23):1911-18.

9. Nakagawa TA, et al. Guidelines for the determination of brain death in infants and children: an update of the 1987 task force recommendations executive summary. Ann Neurol. 2012;71(4):573 85.

Index